D1559525

WHAT EVERY PATIENT, FAMILY, FRIEND, AND CAREGIVER NEEDS TO KNOW ABOUT PSYCHIATRY

WHAT EVERY PATIENT, FAMILY, FRIEND, AND CAREGIVER NEEDS TO KNOW ABOUT PSYCHIATRY

Richard W. Roukema, M.D.

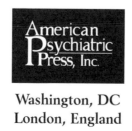

Washington, DC
London, England

Note: The author has worked to ensure that all information in this book concerning drug dosages, schedules, and routes of administration is accurate as of the time of publication and consistent with standards set by the U.S. Food and Drug Administration and the general medical community. As medical research and practice advance, however, therapeutic standards may change. For this reason and because human and mechanical errors sometimes occur, we recommend that readers follow the advice of a physician who is directly involved in their care or the care of a member of their family.

Copyright © 1998 Richard W. Roukema, M.D.
ALL RIGHTS RESERVED
Manufactured in the United States of America on acid-free paper
First Edition   01   00   99   98   4   3   2   1

American Psychiatric Press, Inc.
1400 K Street, N.W., Washington, DC   20005
www.appi.org

Library of Congress Cataloging-in-Publication Data
Roukema, Richard W.
	What every patient, family, friend, and caregiver needs to know about psychiatry / Richard W. Roukema
		p.	cm.
	Includes bibliographical references and index.
	ISBN 0-88048-806-9
	1. Psychiatry—Popular works. 2. Consumer education.
RC460.R68   1998
616.89—dc21
DNLM/DLC   97-31951
for Library of Congress   CIP

British Library Cataloguing in Publication Data
A CIP record is available from the British Library.

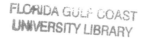

To my family

My wife, Marge
Greg, Susan, Bennett, and Evan
Todd Richard
Jim, Meg, Jimmy, Jenni, and Chris

With love and gratitude

CONTENTS

Foreword xi

PART I

BACKGROUND AND NORMAL VARIATIONS IN STRESS

CHAPTER 1

A Day at the Office 3

CHAPTER 2

Normal Development and the Life Cycle 21

CHAPTER 3

Heredity, Parenting, and Society 35

CHAPTER 4

Stress and Common Emotional Reactions 51

CHAPTER 5

Managing Stress 69

PART II

HOW EMOTIONAL ILLNESS DIFFERS FROM MENTAL ILLNESS

CHAPTER 6

Adjustment Disorders 83

CHAPTER 7

The Neuroses 97

CHAPTER 8

Alcoholism and Drug Abuse 121

CHAPTER 9

Sexual Problems in Our Culture 139

CHAPTER 10

Eating Disorders 163

CHAPTER 11

The Emotional Effects of Loss 183

CHAPTER 12

Personality Disorders 205

CHAPTER 13

Unusual Psychiatric Disorders 223

PART III

MENTAL ILLNESS: THE PSYCHOSES

CHAPTER 14

Mood Disorders: Depression and Manic States . . . 233

CHAPTER 15

Schizophrenic Disorders 253

CHAPTER 16

Other Psychotic Disorders 269

CHAPTER 17

Delirium, Dementia, and Amnestic and
Other Cognitive Disorders 275

PART IV

TREATMENT OF EMOTIONAL AND MENTAL ILLNESSES

CHAPTER 18

How a Psychiatrist Helps 291

CHAPTER 19

Psychotherapy: Who, What, When, and How? . . . 309

CHAPTER 20

Conclusion. 319

Suggested Readings 327

Index 337

Foreword

I remember when I first heard the physician's office and work described as a "cottage industry." I resented the term *industry*, as it hardly pictured the art and practice of medicine as I was living it. There was a time when physicians treated patients. Now physicians are "health care providers," and they treat "consumers" of health care. I am certain that in the future these terms will again be altered.

It takes a while to get used to these changes. Meanwhile, the consumers of health care are becoming much more informed than in the past. No longer is the physician the sole authority on health. Consumers are reading about the latest treatments for virtually all diseases in addition to information from many sources on maintaining health, including alternative medicine. To some, this information must be quite confusing, since there are so many opinions on how best to treat illness and remain healthy and vibrant. But the net result is positive. People seem to be taking more responsibility for their health than ever before.

My patients and their family members have always asked questions about emotional and mental disorders with which they were concerned. In the past, psychiatrists usually had sufficient time to discuss these issues. In today's health maintenance organization setting, however, there is less latitude for patient-physician interaction. To fill this void, much more is being written for the layperson. The latest is *The Merck Manual of Medical Information: Home Edition*, a book for consumers modeled after the well-known *Merck Manual*, long published for the professional.

In the field of mental health, there are books written for the lay reader on specific disorders, but little has been done as an overview of all adult emotional and mental illnesses.

Today's consumers, whether patients, family members, friends, or others giving care to those in distress, need information about these disorders. Beyond this information, caregivers also need some helpful hints on how to care for and help those with whom they work. It is with this goal in mind that I wrote this book.

Other readers, who may not be caregivers, simply may be curious about emotional and mental disorders. For them, I trust that this volume will be informative and hope it is an interesting source of general information on this subject.

I am indebted to Richard Paris for his time and considerable help in editing the first chapter of the manuscript. George Philips, president of Funk and Wagnalls, was kind enough to read my work and encourage me to have it published. His editors, Leon Bram and Richard Eiger, reviewed the book and gave helpful suggestions. My colleagues, Drs. William Layman, Stephen Simring, Richard Frances, Sheldon Miller, and Stephen Schleifer lent early encouragement to my writing. I appreciate and thank those who graciously reviewed the completed book—Drs. Stephen Hyman, Herbert Pardes, and David Kahn. Thanks also to Laurie Flynn and Lucille Joel, who were kind enough to review the book as well. I wish to thank the editors of the American Psychiatric Press, Inc., for their cordial and competent assistance— Carol C. Nadelson, M.D., Editor-in-Chief; Ronald McMillen, Chief Operating Officer; Claire Reinberg, Editorial Director; Pamela Harley, Managing Editor; and Jane Frutchey, Project Editor. Thanks also to my agent, Maryanne Colas, for her enthusiastic support and to my secretary, Judy Van Dyke, for her constant and capable help.

PART I

BACKGROUND

AND

NORMAL VARIATIONS

IN STRESS

CHAPTER 1

A DAY AT THE OFFICE

We all have our days when nothing seems to go right. We all get anxious, fear certain situations, and avoid conflicts. It's part of being alive and human. Some people expect to be happy all the time, and they complain about it when they are not. But such expectations are not realistic. We all experience sadness at some time or another. Loss is common to everyone and must be endured. Stress is familiar to us; it is our constant companion, and it must be handled in appropriate ways in order to prevent anxiety. Dealing with these everyday situations is part of life.

Most of us handle the normal stresses without experiencing too much anxiety, depression, or physical stress. But many exceptions exist. A man or woman may work at the same job for many years and never complain about the stress that is encountered each day. Then suddenly, something happens that is out of the ordinary and it overwhelms the individual. Just such a situation happened to Jill. She was a successful 45-year-old accountant. No stress at work had ever been too much for her. Then one day her boss asked her to go to court to testify about some records that the company had maintained. She was simply required to report on work that the company had done in the past. Jill's own work was not being questioned. She only had to report on some accounting figures. She was not going to be cross-examined or held responsible for any of the documents. Yet, her reaction to this new problem was overwhelming. Jill became anxious and depressed. She could not sleep through the night. Her days were filled with worry and concern about the court appearance. Jill began to worry about whether she was losing control and maybe even losing her mind. She required only a short period of counseling and medication to gain control of her feelings. After the court appearance was over, she resumed her normal activities and was no longer under stress.

Temporary excesses in stress are common. We all have times when our lives can be touched by excessive anxiety. No one escapes an occasional anxious time. Some are able to take stress and anxiety in stride and require no outside assistance. Many people are able to deal better with stress and anxiety by using various self-help methods such as exercise, yoga, and relaxation techniques. Others suffer more and may need help from mental health specialists. Such help is available from many sources, from self-help groups to psychotherapists. A psychiatrist can help to distinguish between the stress that is common to all and the more intense symptoms that require psychiatric treatment. In addition, a psychiatrist is helpful in carefully prescribing medications. In more severe situations, individuals may need admission to psychiatric units in general hospitals or psychiatric hospitals. But it has not always been so. Psychiatrists, psychologists, social workers, and other counselors are a 20th-century phenomenon. They were hardly known in the last century.

In ancient times, mental and emotional illnesses were viewed by most individuals as rooted in a spiritual problem, which required a spiritual solution. The local clergy, with their religious customs, prayers, and rituals, were consulted for assistance. Consulting with clergy also occurred during the Middle Ages. But those afflicted with mental illness, who were regarded as insane, were treated poorly; they were excluded from society and placed in dungeons. Much later, during the American Revolution, Dr. Benjamin Rush treated mentally ill patients more humanely in a hospital in Philadelphia.

From his written record, it is clear that he had a firm grasp on what mental illness was about; he understood and described the behavior and thoughts of the mentally ill very well. Treatments, however, were quite primitive. Bloodletting, purgatives to rid the body of "poisons," and ice-water baths for shock effect were in common use. Still later, during the 19th century, each state built hospitals for the care of the mentally ill. Many of these institutions still remain today, although the population in them has been remarkably reduced.

Meanwhile, the everyday problems that most people experienced were worked out either with home remedies or help from family members, a friend, the clergy, or a local physician. At the time, a severe stigma about mental illness existed. People were expected to either handle their own problems and deal with their own stress or receive minimal help from those around them. Any sign of mental illness in a person was perceived by others with extreme fear, or the person was avoided or ridiculed. Although these attitudes were prevalent in the past, such stigma still remains despite vast improvements in the field of mental health.

The era of modern psychiatry did not begin until the latter part of the 19th century. It was at that time that Sigmund Freud came to the conclusion that illnesses such as anxiety, hysteria, and emotionally induced paralysis of muscles were caused by mental conflicts and that bringing these issues into the patient's awareness helped eliminate symptoms of these neurotic conditions. Through his work and that of his followers, the modern era of psychoanalysis and psychotherapy began.

Much later, another important development occurred. During the early 1950s, new medications were produced through research for the active treatment of the major mental disorders such as schizophrenia and manic depression. This was the beginning of a biological revolution in the field of psychiatry. No longer were physicians helpless in treating these disorders. It led the way to the treatment of mental and emotional illnesses by means of medication and counseling. The modern psychiatrist during that time had a wide array of therapies from which to choose for the care of his or her patients.

Common Questions

Psychiatrists caring for the emotionally and mentally ill are asked many questions about the caregiving done by family members and friends. Among the typical questions that are asked are, "What do I do when my wife becomes panicky?" "Should I push my husband to go to work even when he is depressed?" "What do I say when my elderly mother thinks someone has stolen her shoes, when she has forgotten where she has placed them?" Someone else might ask how to manage the strange behavior of the relative who is schizophrenic but living at home. Such questions are asked by relatives, friends, and others who are on the front lines—those who are trying hard to deal with the emotionally and mentally ill. Teachers, clergy, and various health care workers often are not knowledgeable and secure enough to feel that they are doing the "right thing" in handling the distressed person. Such concerned and involved persons want to be helpful. They often worry about whether their communications and actions are really going to assist the person in need or be detrimental. Although information alone often is not sufficient to assist those who are in contact with the emotionally or mentally ill, knowledge about such illnesses can be a basis or starting point for dealing with distressed individuals. For example, dealing with an alcoholic person may be confusing and frustrating if one is not familiar with the disease. But the information obtained by a member in Alcoholics Anonymous or by the family member in Al-Anon can be extremely helpful in dealing with an alcoholic relative. Similarly, some familiarity with mental and emotional disorders is useful to those who are dealing with these problems on a daily basis.

It is not unusual for an individual to request a consultation with a psychiatrist about a particular problem that is mild or just in its early stages (e.g., "I just wanted to check it out to see if I am on the right track."). Some problems are not serious and may require only one or two sessions to resolve. Not everyone needs a prolonged period of psychoanalysis or medication for his or her distress. But there are difficulties in living that people experience that are not so easily dismissed.

In this book, both the common stresses of everyday life and the more complicated psychiatric problems that are seen in the psychiatrist's office are discussed. Whenever possible, useful suggestions are given for each disorder to help patients and their relatives or other caregivers in understanding the nature of the difficulties that they may encounter and how to deal with them.

The next discussion is an overview of the typical problems that are brought to the consulting room of the psychiatrist. The illnesses and concerns presented are common to patients and are seen every day by psychiatrists, who are engaged in private practice or working in clinics throughout the country.

Common Problems in Psychiatry

Case Example

It happened all at once. When she least expected it, Anne became extremely anxious and upset. She was enjoying herself at a concert in New York City, listening attentively to the orchestra. Suddenly she experienced a profound physical sensation. It was difficult to breathe, her heart was pounding, and she felt weak and was certain that she would faint. Her head began to spin and she felt completely out of control. She knew that she had to get out of the concert hall at once. Anne tugged at her husband's arm and told him that she had to leave. He was surprised by her insistence, as he had no idea that she was having a panic reaction. They left the hall and started for home. As they were traveling up the West Side Highway toward the George Washington Bridge, Anne began to feel better, but she still felt weak and anxious. Upon arriving home, she immediately poured herself a few ounces of vodka to alleviate her tension. The next day she called her physician and made an appointment. He examined her and found her to be in good physical condition, although her pulse was slightly elevated. He assured her that she was in fine health and that her symptoms were due to anxiety. Anne felt momentarily satisfied but worried that the "attack" would come back.

Several days later, while out shopping at a supermarket, Anne had another episode. It was a repetition of the same distressing feelings, only worse. This time she thought she would lose her mind. She rested at the market for a while and then went home. Anne called her physician and told him the news. He asked her to come into his office again. The physician found nothing that indicated any physical disease and suggested that she call a psychiatrist.

The very word *psychiatrist* brought to mind other worries. Anne wondered, Am I going to have the same problem that my uncle had? He was in a mental hospital for years. Is this the way it begins? Now she became even more anxious. Anne called her husband at work, told him about her visit to the physician, and asked him what to do. When he became aware of her fear and anxiety, he told her that he would be home shortly and would arrange to take her to a psychiatrist. The road to my office seemed long. The anxiety did not dissipate at all during the ride. But shortly after Anne arrived at my office, she asked the questions that were most on her mind: "Doctor, am I going crazy? Am I going to have to go to a mental hospital?" After hearing about the symptoms, it was apparent to me that she was suffering from a typical panic disorder. I assured her that she was not going crazy and that I had never seen anyone become insane following symptoms such as she was experiencing. When she heard this statement, she felt immediate relief and began to relax. But the next question was, "Will it come back?" I informed her that such symptoms may recur but that there are good medications that can help alleviate the symptoms and prevent attacks from returning. I also told her that we should meet again to investigate the possible origin of her panic attacks. She agreed to do so and treatment began.

Phobic Disorders

For reasons that are unclear, phobias have become prevalent in today's culture. These abnormal fears are present in a high percentage of the population. Many people simply avoid the feared object or situation and thus never ask for treatment for their phobias (e.g., elevators, escalators, snakes). Others rationalize their phobias.

Someone who is afraid to fly can say that his or her friends are stupid for flying because it is dangerous. But some phobias can be disabling, particularly if they interfere with a person's vocation. For example, if a truck driver suddenly develops a phobia about driving, it has more significance than it would have for someone who is not dependent on driving for his or her economic well-being. Phobias sometimes disappear spontaneously; others remain for a lifetime.

As a response to the increase of phobias in our culture, phobia clinics have been established in most major cities in this country. In addition, psychiatrists and other psychotherapists treat many patients with phobias, and they do so successfully. New treatments using medication and behavioral techniques have largely replaced the traditional use of psychoanalysis, although in some cases psychoanalysis is still a good long-term approach to the problem of phobic symptoms.

Mood Disorders

Changes in mood come on suddenly or gradually and are upsetting. Perhaps you know of a friend or relative who has experienced acute depression. You may have witnessed the profound lack of energy, the loss of appetite, the difficulty sleeping, the feelings of despair, and even the rumination about suicide. It makes the onlooker feel helpless. The following is a typical case example illustrating depression:

Case Example

One day, a 55-year-old executive came to see me because of a dramatic change in his mood; he was markedly depressed. A few weeks before, Bill was making major decisions in his position with a large Fortune 500 company. Bill wondered how this could happen to him. Wasn't he a dynamic personality? How could he suddenly become so depressed that he could not make even small decisions anymore? His appetite had all but disappeared, and sleep was almost impossible. His mood was hopeless; he won-

dered how he could ever return to work and assume any responsibilities. His family was equally surprised at his condition, as they
had never seen him like this before. It was apparent that he could
do little, although his wife struggled to get him to do some household chores. Even simple tasks were beyond his ability at the time.
The days were long and dreary; suicide was very much on Bill's
mind.

At the suggestion of a friend, Bill's wife made an appointment
to see me at my office. Bill did not want to come, but at his wife's
insistence, he reluctantly came for a consultation. It was apparent
that Bill was suffering from a serious depression and needed immediate treatment. Because of his suicidal ideas, it was necessary
for me to hospitalize him in a psychiatric unit of a general hospital,
where he could be given appropriate medication and could be
watched for changes in his condition. He reluctantly accepted my
recommendation that he be hospitalized. At first, he remained depressed and unable to do anything to help himself, but gradually he
began to respond. In 3 weeks, he was well enough to go home on
a maintenance dose of medication. Within 2 months, he was back
to work part-time, and in another month, he was fully functional.

Such cases of depression are common. They can happen to anyone. They are serious and can be brought on by external problems or
for no apparent reason at all. In the last 30 years, psychiatry has made
great strides in dealing with depression, with more success during
this short period of time than in all previous centuries.

Some individuals who suffer from depression also have times
when they feel unusually well, have an enormous amount of energy,
and feel "high." Frequently, while consulting with someone in my
office, I have been asked, "Do my mood swings mean that I am
a manic-depressive?" This is an important question, particularly if
there is a history of such illness in the family. It is essential for the psychiatrist to distinguish between day-to-day fluctuations in mood that
are common and within normal limits and the massive mood swings
seen in patients with manic-depressive disorder (now called bipolar
disorder). This illness has been researched extensively and has been
found to be inherited and have a biological basis. In the past, many
patients with bipolar disorder had to be hospitalized for long periods

of time. Now the devastating effects of this disorder controlled successfully in a high percentage of patients with the use of lithium and other medications.

Drugs and Alcohol

Many patients have questions about the disease of alcoholism. "Is alcoholism inherited?" "My father was an alcoholic. Does this mean that I am more likely to become an alcoholic?" "If I drink alcohol, will my children be more likely to drink?" "Can you become an alcoholic if you only drink beer?" "Why doesn't my husband realize that he is an alcoholic when it is so obvious to everyone else?" Most psychiatrists are able to answer these questions well.

It has taken the general physician a long time to admit to the tragedy that results from the excessive use of alcohol. The deaths caused by driving under the influence of alcohol are well known. Diseases such as cirrhosis of the liver, inflammation of the pancreas, withdrawal reactions (delirium tremens), and certain forms of heart disease are also the result of excessive alcohol use. Although physicians have known that these conditions are caused by alcohol, there has been, in the past, a reluctance to confront the alcoholic person with his or her illness. The more recent acceptance of alcoholism as a "disease" rather than just a bad habit has done much to point the way toward a rehabilitation and treatment program for alcoholic patients. The combination of medical treatment and Alcoholics Anonymous is effective in dealing with alcoholism.

During the first half of this century, the use of mind-altering drugs was confined to the inner city and to certain artists and performers. But in the last 30 years, there has been an epidemic of drug use by teenagers and young adults, which has taken its toll in illness and premature deaths. The public has been assaulted with information in the media; at times it has been confusing.

Currently, much more is known about the effects of "street drugs" on physical and mental health and how these drugs interfere with the ability to function well. New treatments have evolved, and the importance of self-help groups such as Alcoholics Anonymous and Narcotics Anonymous cannot be overemphasized.

Questions about the use of prescribed medications are asked frequently by patients. "Will taking a drug make me dependent on it? Will I be able to get off it or will I have withdrawal effects?" It has been my experience that when someone is that concerned about the problem of drug dependence, the psychiatrist does not have to worry about that person becoming dependent or addicted. Rather, such individuals have to be encouraged to take enough of the medication to be effective, since such persons are so afraid of addiction that they tend to skip doses. It is important that each patient use enough of a prescribed medication so that its effectiveness can be maximized.

Changes in Marriage

Marriage problems appear to be increasing in our society. When I first began my practice some years ago, I read a book entitled *Neurotic Interaction in Marriage*. It highlighted the fact that individuals are attracted to each other for conscious as well as unconscious reasons. For example, it is not unusual for a quiet, shy, and introverted person to be attracted to a talkative extroverted individual. In such an instance, each person sees in the other traits not possessed by the self. But these attractions are not always recognized consciously when the two individuals first meet. The attraction occurs nevertheless. Probably no marriage exists without a degree of "neurotic" involvement between the partners. It is generally outside one's awareness. This is not to say that it is abnormal. Rather, it is one of the reasons why attraction, infatuation, and love are so powerful. To a large extent, this involvement is healthy and is of no concern to the psychotherapist. But when the neurotic interaction is intense, it can sometimes become destructive.

Marriage has proven to be a difficult institution; less than half of the population appear to manage it at all. Perhaps only one-third of marriages really function well. Furthermore, the expectations of the partners in marriage have changed over the years, and the commitment to marriage has been altered remarkably. Many people come to psychiatrists or other psychotherapists for counseling about marriage problems. Some ask how to change the other person. Others want to know how to change themselves in order to adjust to the other person. If the marriage partners are genuinely motivated to remain married and are committed to improving their relationship, much can be done to facilitate the process and make the marriage work.

Problems Common to the Elderly

There are a number of physical disorders that bring on mental symptoms; these are seen most commonly among the elderly. For example, a patient may have a sudden onset of dizziness, disorientation, difficulty remembering things, and a general loss of control. These symptoms may last a short time and gradually clear up. They are disturbing to patients, and the patients may feel that they are "going crazy." Usually this is due to a circulatory problem and may portend more serious symptoms in the future such as a cerebral hemorrhage or thrombosis resulting in a stroke. Frequently, however, patients have only one episode and can live quite well for years without further difficulty.

Case Example

One day, I was called into the local hospital to see an elderly woman. Sarah had been admitted for an abdominal condition, and she had been functioning well mentally before her admission. The evening after she had come to the hospital, she began to have symptoms that were frightening to her. She became markedly disoriented; she thought she was in her childhood home. She called for her mother who had long since died. She misidentified the nurses as her sisters and even had trouble calling her husband by name. Sarah's memory was impaired, and she was extremely anxious. She did not remember my name and appeared to confuse me with someone else. She gave her full name correctly but could not name the hospital, even though she had been quite familiar with it. Her husband could not comprehend the changes that had occurred in such a short time. But after only 2 days of care and appropriate medication, her condition began to stabilize, and within 2 more days, she was mentally healthy again.

As in this example, some types of acute organic psychoses can come and go quickly. But to the patient and the family, these events are distressing.

Fear of Mental Illness

Many people have trouble making up their minds about things. Every day, we all have to decide on small or large issues. Some individuals can make decisions instantly and seem to have few regrets about their decisions. Others, by contrast, appear to be ambivalent about many issues. Fred was such a person.

Case Example

Fred obsessed about everything. No decision seemed easy for him. One day he was bothered by conflicting feelings about his wife. He said that some days he loved her very much, but other days he could not stand the sight of her, although he would never tell her how he felt. On a particular day when he was in my office, he appeared unusually worried. After much hesitation about the subject, he revealed his concern. "I can never make up my mind about things. I don't even feel the same about my wife from one day to the other. Am I a 'split personality'?" It was not hard to guess the next question: "Am I a schizophrenic?"

Many individuals confuse the two terms *split personality* and *schizophrenia*. They are not at all the same condition. Schizophrenia is a severe mental illness in which various functions of the mind are affected to some degree, while other areas remain intact. For example, the patient may be clearly oriented as to the current date, time, location, and his or her identity and have a disturbance in thinking that makes his or her ideas vague and unclear. Or the patient may be delusional, as in paranoia. He or she may hear voices that others do not hear. Split personality, by contrast, is an illness in which multiple personalities are manifested at different times, as in the movie *The Three Faces of Eve*. It is a rare and often debilitating illness. Fred was not suffering from either of these disorders. Rather, he had difficulty making up his mind to a greater degree than most individuals. The reason for this was explored in psychotherapy. A psychiatrist can help clarify the doubts and fears about severe illness, such as Fred had, thereby alleviating the patient's anxiety.

The Psychoses

Some individuals are unfortunate enough to have the most troubling of all psychiatric illnesses. This group of disorders is generally referred to as the psychoses. Illnesses such as schizophrenia, manic-depressive disorder (bipolar disorder), paranoid disorders, brief psychotic reactions, and others are extremely disturbing to patients and family alike. To lose control of one's thinking processes, to be unable to react appropriately to social and work situations, to perceive what others do not see or hear, and to be unable to react emotionally to others are symptoms typical of psychoses and are truly the most difficult experiences that any human being can endure. Probably the worst of these illnesses is known as schizophrenia. About 1% of the population develops this form of mental illness at some time. It is debilitating in its effect on personality, performance, thought processes, and emotional reactions of the persons involved. Some forms of schizophrenia come on suddenly; others come on slowly and insidiously. There are acute manifestations and more chronic forms. Some patients are docile, but others are extremely active and can create major disturbances in families and in the community. Regardless of the type of schizophrenia, there are far more effective treatments available now than at any time in the past. Antipsychotic medications now used in the treatment of the psychoses diminish the emotional pain that patients must suffer.

Research on medications to treat the major psychiatric illnesses has increased greatly during the last 30 years. The biochemistry of the brain is becoming increasingly clear, although brain research is still at a primitive stage compared to what is expected in the next 50–100 years. Many medications have been developed, and each year newer drugs appear for management of the major psychoses and other psychiatric illnesses. Researchers hope they eventually will find cures for these disorders.

Multiple Symptoms

Sexual difficulties, reactions to loss, personality disorders, and behavioral quirks are commonly seen by psychiatrists. Occasionally, some or all of these problems can occur within the same person.

Case Example

Some time ago, a young, recently married man, Jack, consulted me about premature ejaculation, which is a common sexual difficulty among young males. He wanted specific help with this functional difficulty, but at the same time he spoke of his terrible feelings of loss. He felt that his manhood was diminished, that his wife would no longer respect him, and that she would divorce him. These feelings resulted in a degree of depression. He wondered if he were strange and unusual. He asked if he was the only one to have such a difficulty. Was it a personality problem? Was he losing control or losing his mind? Such thoughts troubled him constantly. I assured Jack that of all the sexual difficulties that can befall men, premature ejaculation is probably the easiest to treat, if the person comes for help early. I also assured him that the doubts and fears that he had were temporary side effects of his primary concern—the sexual dysfunction. After about 6 months of psychotherapy, he was functioning well sexually, had regained his self-respect, and was not troubled by his thoughts.

The loss of the ability to perform sexually is one form of loss, but losses can be experienced in many ways.

Other Losses

Human beings are subject to a variety of losses, such as the loss of loved ones and the loss of prestige, position, financial security, and one's job. People react to such losses in many ways. Some handle the losses with dispatch; others mourn losses and are depressed for months or years; still others deal with loss by the excessive use of alcohol or other drugs. There are persons who resort to suicide, thus ending the torture of depression, helplessness, and low self-esteem. However, most people handle loss with mild reactions of mourning, depression, insomnia, and anxiety. These symptoms usually disappear in time. Many people consult clergy, friends, or self-help groups when dealing with loss. When an extreme reaction to loss occurs, it is a good time to seek help from a psychiatrist.

Personality Disorders

People with personality disorders do not often seek help from psychiatrists. They usually are not bothered by their particular personality traits, but these same traits often present difficulty for people around them. For example, an individual with a paranoid personality is generally a quarrelsome, doubting, suspicious person. Yet, he or she will seldom go to a psychiatrist for help. The schizoid person is quiet and withdrawn, is given to much daydreaming and fantasy, and has poor interpersonal relationships. Such an individual will hardly ever seek counseling on his or her own, even though the need for therapy may seem obvious to friends and relatives. Similarly, the aggressive or the narcissistic person rarely seeks out assistance from a psychotherapist.

Individuals with these personality types create much anguish and distress in others. As a result, the psychiatrist often will see the husband or wife of the individual who has the personality problem, since it is the family member who all too frequently becomes the object of the peculiar behavior of the person who has a personality disorder.

The relative may ask, "How do I handle him when he does these outrageous things?" "What do I do with her when she withdraws and does not want to talk to me or see anyone?" Personality differences are often the source of problems in families and in the workplace.

Modern Stress

Many persons are concerned about the general problem of anxiety and how to cope with the increasing stresses of modern society. It has been said that this is the age of anxiety. It is difficult to know whether living today is any more stressful than it was 100 years ago or at any time in history. We tend to romanticize the past and think of it only in favorable terms. But when only a little thought is given to the distant past, it is not hard to imagine the physical price that was demanded of humans on a daily basis just for them to stay alive. They had to carry water from the well, use the outhouse, wash clothes by hand, read by candlelight or gas lamp, ride a horse or a carriage, eat with little variety in menu, and work 10–12 hours a day at hard physical labor. Many children died in infancy; mothers frequently died during or shortly after childbirth. And many people of all ages died of infections, although today this is a rare occurrence. I really do not think that life was easier in the good old days. Nor was it less stressful in an emotional sense. But there was one significant difference: everybody was forced to exercise their muscles whether they wished to do so or not. In order to survive, people had to do much more than push buttons. Using the large muscles of the body may well have drained away much of the anxiety that was consciously felt by people. Now we resort to jogging, swimming, walking, or some other form of exercise to compensate for the loss of such activity, all of which occurred as a by-product of civilization.

A certain amount of anxiety is normal, but excessive anxiety is an abnormal state of arousal. It has all of the physical ingredients of a readiness to fight or run away. Exercise will partially relieve anxiety, but it is up to the person to try to deal with the causes of his or her excessive anxiety. Most often, anxiety is due to emotional problems, but sometimes the cause is due to a physical disease such as hyperthyroidism or hypoglycemia. If the origin is physical, it must be handled by a physician familiar with the particular physical problem. If the cause appears to be due to stress and emotional factors, help can be obtained sometimes through self-help books or organizations; often, the help must be obtained through consultation with a mental health professional.

Stress and its various manifestations can lead to psychosomatic problems. Many physical diseases are greatly influenced by stress. Ailments such as headaches, stomach ulcers, colitis, thyroid disease, asthma, and neurodermatitis are worsened or even caused by stress. The same can be said of pain. Regardless of the origin of pain, even if it is caused by organic factors, the presence of stress tends to increase the amount and frequency of pain.

Changes?

Has the overall incidence of emotional and mental problems increased in modern times? This is difficult to answer definitively. Certainly, we know more about these illnesses now than in the past and can do more about them. It is a common observation among physicians that as new treatments are found for an illness, many more patients are discovered for treatment for that illness. This finding was noted particularly with the discovery of lithium for the treatment of bipolar disorder, antidepressants for depression, and medications and behavior modification for panic disorders.

Despite the improved treatments available, much mystery, mythology, and confusion remain about the field of psychiatry. There is still considerable stigma and fear about emotional and mental illnesses, although among the general public, there are signs that more understanding and acceptance are in fact occurring and that the stigma regarding these illnesses is decreasing.

Overview

The purpose of this book is to help readers differentiate between the normal range of stresses and anxieties that are common to us all and the types of illnesses that can occur and are seen in the day-to-day experience of any psychiatrist. With a basic knowledge of the field of psychiatry, the parent, husband, wife, or other family member, as well as the teacher, health care worker, clergyperson, or police officer—those on the front lines—will be better equipped to deal with, in an understanding way, the emotionally or mentally disturbed person. Patients will be able to benefit from knowledge of these illnesses as well. Although the information provided is generally accepted by the majority of psychiatrists in this country, it should be borne in mind that the field is continually changing as new discoveries are made.

In succeeding chapters in this book, I describe normal development in general, hereditary considerations, parenting, and the current impact of society on human development. I also discuss the subject of daily stresses as experienced by many of us and suggest how to cope with these stresses. A major focus of this book is specific psychiatric disorders that are seen in the psychiatrist's consulting room and how they are treated.

Throughout the book, I present a number of observations on various subjects based on my personal reflections. These observations are not to be regarded as absolute fact. Changes that have occurred in the treatment of various disorders over the years are acknowledged.

Suggested readings, organized by chapter, are provided at the end of this book so that readers can gather more details about a given subject if desired.

CHAPTER 2

NORMAL DEVELOPMENT AND THE LIFE CYCLE

When my children were growing up, I was in awe of the rapid changes in their growth, the sudden discoveries of newfound abilities, and the dramatic alterations in their emotional development. From their complete dependence at birth, to lively interaction throughout infancy, to seeking out partial independence as toddlers, they, like all children, were a marvel to behold. The careful negotiating of a step, the demand for food or care, the first assertive "no," and the joy of play in any form—these are some of the many things that I remember fondly.

At present, I am living through another part of the life cycle, as a grandfather. Watching my grandchildren is even more fascinating. To update my grandchildren's parents, I visited several bookstores for the latest information on child care.

The bookstores that I frequent are filled with new information on child development and child care. Unlike a few generations ago, when books by Spock and Gesell were the only sources that parents had to consult, today's parents have an abundance of books to read. If you have children or grandchildren, you will recognize the different stages of development that I summarize in this chapter. This information is taken from various authorities in the field of child development. I have not tried to cover every theory but have chosen what stands out in my experience as important. For greater detail, I suggest reading more information about this interesting topic.

Overview of Human Development

Normal human development occurs in two ways, depending on how one views the subject. From one view, it consists of continuous development beginning in childhood when the developing person proceeds along a preordained path common to all. One step follows upon another in well-defined ways. Freud's psychosexual stages and Erikson's eight stages of man fit into this category. From another view, development appears to occur in spurts, with occasional regressions. In some individuals, there is no forward movement in their development, and they may remain fixed psychologically at a particular stage. But it is also possible that growth left unfinished in a previous stage is accomplished partially in succeeding stages. Thus, some developmental stages are never fully achieved, and others are delayed but eventually reached. Both views are useful to consider in studying normal growth and development.

Many studies have been done by pediatricians, psychologists, and psychiatrists to help define what happens in the growing child. Biological growth in terms of size, neurological change, and motor development has been measured. Normal ranges for all these areas of development have been described. Endocrinological, psychological, and cognitive development also has been studied. Even the typical development of language and morality in the growing child has been observed and delineated.

Before modern times, human development was taken for granted. Even if babies survived birth, many did not live through the first year. If they were fortunate, they grew up to become adults. Infections from accidents or epidemics took the lives of the young. Unlike today, childhood ended early, at age 11 or 12 years, or younger, at which time the child was expected to begin working to help the adults cope with the immense amount of physical work necessary for survival. The prolonged adolescence that we now permit is a modern invention. With affluence and the need for more education, whether technical or academic, the young have become more dependent on their families, thus extending adolescence for many years. Some young people do not begin to contribute toward their own support until they are in their late 20s or early 30s.

During the 19th century, there was little interest in the early development of the child from infancy to adulthood. No one seemed concerned with pursuing such a course. It was not until the last part of the 19th century that Freud began to talk about the different stages of development.

Freud's Psychosexual Stages

Sigmund Freud was perhaps the first person to attempt to delineate in a systematic way the stages through which the child passes. He was concerned with the biological events of childhood and the corresponding emotional changes in the developing child. From his studies of the neurotic adult, he theorized stages of development through which each child passes. Furthermore, he postulated that if a child remained too long at any one stage, his or her character and emotional life would be altered or inhibited in terms of the future. For example, fixation at the oral stage of a child's development could result in excessive dependency on others, and fixation at the anal stage could bring about obsessive-compulsive behavior.

The *oral stage* begins at birth, when the infant has already acquired the need to suck and turn its head (rooting reflex) in the direction of the source of food. Without such an obvious instinctual move, the child would not survive. But with it comes the closeness of the infant to the mother. The child is fed, and simultaneously the mother is helping the child develop psychologically. Holding, caressing, rocking, and talking to the child are of enormous importance in the child's development. Studies of children in orphanages, where care by adults was extremely limited, have shown that children who are not attended to emotionally and are not picked up, caressed, and held appear to become withdrawn and depressed. Some have died, even though no observable physical disease was present.

The regular and sufficient supply of food to the infant, along with the necessary nurturing, gives the newborn the security that he or she needs. If something interferes with the normal process in this stage, an arrest in development occurs. Thereafter, the child may be concerned excessively with satisfying oral needs, both physically and emotionally. As a result, conditions such as obesity, anorexia, or bulimia may follow in adolescence or adult life. If the conflict over the satisfaction of needs is mild, there may be some compensation made in later stages. But if the problem is severe, pathology results. Oral fixation and excessive dependency on others may occur in adult life.

The *anal stage* begins at about 18–24 months. It centers around bowel training. It is the time when the child is able to protest and say no to parental wishes. If the parent is concerned with early bowel training, the child may resist and conflict will result. The child can withhold his or her feces, play with them, appear to regard them as his or her possession, and not part with them easily. For some parents, especially the more fastidious, this is cause for concern, whereas other parents deal with such matters more casually. Some children pass through this stage easily. Others take considerable time to do so, even when parents have successfully worked through this stage with siblings. I have seen children who were still soiling their pants at age 6 or 7 years because of a failure to negotiate this stage successfully. This behavior is clearly abnormal. I have known parents who delayed bowel training up to ages 4 and 5 years with the permissive view that the child will use the toilet for bowel movements when he or she is ready. During my psychoanalytic training, I reported such an example in delay of bowel training by a mother, whose 5-year-old child had not yet been trained. My Viennese-born supervisor responded with alarm, "When do these parents expect ego development to begin?"

Freud stated in his writings that fixation at the anal stage of development resulted in the adult being excessively concerned about money, time, dirt, and germs. He maintained that traits such as obstinacy, miserliness, and orderliness develop and form the obsessive-compulsive personality.

The *phallic stage* begins at about age 3 years. At that time, the child becomes increasingly interested in the genital area. Freud spoke mainly about male interest in the penis and the child's fascination with the pleasure that he experiences in manipulating the genital area. He postulated that some male children developed *castration anxiety* and fear during this period and that females were subject to *penis envy*, or envy of what the male child can do. There was little scientific basis for Freud's conclusions, but the theories about early sexuality have remained in the psychiatric literature as authentic dogma. To some psychiatrists, castration anxiety and penis envy are seen not as actual problems for children but more as metaphors or symbols for what happens emotionally during these periods.

During the phallic stage, the male child wishes the exclusive attention of the mother to the exclusion of the father, thus ushering in the *oedipal stage* of psychosexual development. The healthy male child negotiates this stage by gradually identifying with his father and taking on the father's values as his own. If the male child remains attached to his mother too long and identifies with her too much, neurotic conflicts and problems in character development may occur.

The *latency stage* follows at about age 7 years and continues until puberty. Freud believed that during the latency stage, the child was less concerned with sexual matters and more involved with mastering his or her environment and with games, toys, school, and peers. This involvement occurs, according to Freud, because of the child's fear of castration and his or her repression of sexual desires. Although children are preoccupied with these other activities, few psychiatrists now believe that sexual interests are truly placed on the back burner at this time. Children during this stage are curious and play various exploratory games such as "doctor" and mutual masturbation.

Finally, with the onset of puberty, the *genital stage* arrives. Genital gratification becomes of prime importance. During this stage, the parents of the child recede into the background and assume less importance, while peers become the main focus of attention. The stage is now set for the active pursuit of sexual "objects" and the eventual development of mature sexual responses and relationships. Freud did not go on to describe other stages of the life cycle. He believed that the early stages set the way for future character traits and behavior and that adults repeated in a compulsive way the patterns laid down in childhood in what Freud called the *repetition-compulsion.*

Freud's developmental scheme is based on a biological form of relatedness, on the fulfillment of biological needs. Later, other psychoanalysts (Abraham, Horney, Sullivan, Fromm, and others) stressed the emotional interactions that occur between the child and the significant persons in his or her life. They believed that such relationships were far more important than the specific psychosexual events that occurred at any given stage. They called attention to the importance of the child's culture and education and to the influence of his or her peers, teachers, and other environmental factors. Thus, they did not adhere to Freud's biological basis of child development but were more impressed by the multitude of factors that influenced a child's development.

Erikson's Eight Stages of Man

The well-known psychologist and psychoanalyst Erik Erikson provided a broader and more enlightened view of how children developed at various stages. He enlarged on Freud's biological approach with a more inclusive description of the stages of man throughout life. He related the biological instincts to the psychological factors occurring at the various stages. Erikson emphasized the parental, social, and moral influences that affect the individual. He felt that it was important for the developing person to manage certain tasks successfully at each stage in order to go on to the next stage.

Erikson first postulated the *oral-sensory stage: trust versus mistrust/hope.* During this stage, the child's behavior consists mostly of incorporating things. The infant takes in food orally and with his or her eyes and other senses takes in information from the environment. If the caregiver of the child regularly provides proper nourishment and adequate physical and emotional care, the child will develop a basic feeling of trust. Erikson states that it is equally important for the infant to learn to mistrust those around him or her who do not provide the basic needs or who appear to do him or her harm. Later, the perceived balance between trust and mistrust develops into a crucial ability to discern between those peers and adults who seek the child's best interest and those who are out to do physical or emotional harm. Thus, Erikson provides a psychosocial dimension that builds on Freud's original concept of the oral stage of psychosexual development.

From the basic trust-mistrust relationship that evolves in the early stage of life comes the virtue of hope. Everyone is familiar with the saying, Hope springs eternal in the human breast. Erikson postulates that hope has its origin in the oral-sensory stage of life. It is the expectation that good things are ahead, that needs will be met, and that life will be satisfying. That trait is very human—the hope that exists even in the most devastating circumstances such as in concentration camps or in the presence of severe illness. It has always been amazing to me how hope can exist in people who are going through such extreme trauma. Only in the case of clinical depression does hope sometimes disappear entirely.

In speaking of hope as a virtue, Erikson theorizes the origin of other virtues such as industry, purpose, and will, qualities that are seldom referred to in the writings of psychiatrists and psychoanalysts. Reference to such virtues is one of the unique contributions of Erikson's approach to child development.

During the second and third years of life, the child reaches the *muscular-anal stage: autonomy versus shame/doubt.* He or she gains mobility and simultaneously begins to have a sense of purpose. In watching my grandchildren at this stage, I have commented to my wife, "They have their agenda." There are goals in mind that are pursued one after the other. Erikson says that this is the stage in which the child's will becomes manifested. As a result, there is a battle between the will of the child and that of the parents. Thus, the legendary "terrible twos" about which new parents are warned. Theoretically, if children are excessively controlled at this stage, they may doubt their own will, doubt their abilities, feel shame, and develop an exaggerated conformity to those around them. On the other hand, failure to control some children's impulses at this stage may lead to lack of ego control on the part of the children. It is necessary for parents to give children a degree of structure within which they can grow effectively without having their will thwarted excessively. The way to accomplish this goal is the subject of many books on child rearing.

Erikson emphasized that the failure to negotiate successfully any one of these stages may be partially overcome by good relationships and experiences in future stages. Erikson refers to the phallic stage as the *locomotor-genital stage: initiative versus guilt/purpose*. It occurs at about ages 3–5 years. During this time, the male child becomes increasingly interested in his genitals. He is consumed with his ability to move about and to manipulate his environment. He develops initiative and self-motivation. He idealizes his parents, thus setting the stage for his oedipal attachment to his mother. Similarly, the female child develops the above abilities, but she relates adoringly to her father. At this stage, exaggerated guilt on the part of the child of either sex may occur due to conscious or unconscious wishes to be close to one parent. With the introduction of guilt, moral development begins, and a rudimentary conscience is first seen. This oedipal attachment may last inordinately long and prevent normal relationships with peers in adolescence or in adult life. At this stage, the child also develops a greater sense of purpose, a direction and goal toward which he or she strives even in play.

The next stage occurs at age 5 or 6 years and extends to puberty. Erikson called this the *latency stage: industry versus inferiority/competence*. Although there is considerable interest in sexuality during this stage, sexual interests are certainly not as great as they are after puberty. During the latency period, children are absorbed in learning as much as they can about their environment. They attempt to master their surroundings physically and mentally and to become competent to deal with whatever confronts them. Erikson speaks of this stage as a time for industriousness. If children fail to accomplish what they set out to do, they may develop a feeling of inferiority. By contrast, repeated successes generate confidence and enable them to go on to more difficult tasks.

The final stage of psychosexual development proposed by Freud is the genital stage, which occurs after puberty. At this stage, the sexual energy of the adolescent is directed toward someone usually of the opposite sex. Erikson refers to this stage as the *adolescent stage: identity versus role diffusion/fidelity.* It is the task of the adolescent to try on one "mask" after another to see which is to his or her liking. Eventually, the adolescent feels comfortable with one mode of being, with one identity. Simultaneously, he or she develops the virtue of fidelity—the ability to have an allegiance to a particular view or ideology. Identity and fidelity together with the successful passage through the previous stages lead to the formation of a strong sense of self (ego). In Erikson's words, "adolescence is really representative of what each individual's ego strength must tackle at one and the same time, namely, inner unruliness and changing conditions" (Evans 1967, p. 33). Most adolescents are able to meet this inner turmoil and survive quite well. If the individual is not successful in working out these changes and developments, the ego is left weak and confused.

In our relatively free and affluent society, adolescents have an unusual number of choices from which to select their goals. The adolescent's identity is closely connected to the person, group, or activity with which the adolescent identifies. Even two or three generations ago, the choices were relatively few. Previously, one could choose to go from high school to the workplace, to go to college for further education, or to enter military service. Today, there are many more options. Spending up to a year or two traveling, entering a commune, being a ski bum, and living at home with parents are among the many choices that adolescents now make. Without the affluence that is present for many, and the influence of the media, which highlight these opportunities, these possibilities would not exist. Increased choices create more difficulties for adolescent identity formation. But more creative potentials are also possible.

Freud did not extend his psychosexual stages beyond the genital stage (i.e., puberty.) Erikson goes on to describe the *young adult stage: intimacy versus isolation—love.*

As background to Erikson's young adult stage, it is appropriate to mention an observation by an American psychiatrist Harry Stack Sullivan. It was his opinion that at age 5 or 6 years, the child is able gradually to develop a "love" relationship with a friend, usually of the same sex, at a time when he or she can care for and give to another person out of feelings for that individual. Sullivan called this the "chum" stage of development. He felt that this ability to regard a peer as a best friend is essential to the future development of adult intimate relationships. During this early time, the child is able to share his or her possessions and exhibit some concern for the welfare of the other person. I am certain that this stage is quite important for the adult to reach the intimacy necessary for a relationship in adult life. Erikson stressed the idea that true intimacy and love require genuine care and concern for the other person. Often, these qualities supersede the person's own immediate needs, and the identities of the two are somewhat fused toward a common good. Ideally, the identities of both should complement each other to their mutual benefit. If one person's identity is too heavily involved with the other, the relationship may become strained.

To be fully adult, the individual must be able to become intimate with another person and feel and act in a genuinely loving manner. Failure to do so leads one into isolation but does not mean that everyone who is unmarried or not living intimately with another person has not reached this stage successfully. It is quite possible to be loving and caring for others while not living with them. In our society, most individuals choose some form of cohabitation, but there are many single persons who are fully adult, have intimate relationships, and are not isolated. Such arrangements usually involve some form of commitment to the other person.

At Erikson's next stage, *adulthood stage: generativity versus stagnation/care*, the adult contributes to society at large. He or she may produce an idea, create a work of art, raise a family, be inventive, or in some way help the groups or institutions with which he or she is associated. Each person has the potential to generate something within the framework of his or her possibilities. Failure to do this in adult life results in stagnation of development in the person's growth potential. I have seen individuals who showed no further emotional or intellectual growth after their early 20s. Some in their 40s seem to have lived their lives as fully as they ever will, reaching stagnation in the mid-life stage. In contrast, some active persons continue their productivity well into old age. Erikson himself was a good example of the latter type of person.

The concept of caring for others, including friends, family, the environment, or the world at large, requires a degree of maturity and generativity. Such caring provides the cement that holds together the various elements of society.

Erikson's final stage, *old age and maturity stage: ego integrity versus despair/wisdom,* focuses on the ability of the ego to gather together the experiences and accomplishments of the past into a satisfactory whole. The person in old age reflects on the past with a degree of wisdom that was not present to the same extent before this stage. This wisdom does not happen to everyone; it is an ideal. Many persons fall into despair and fret about the lack of ability to do the things that were possible in youth. Regrets, worries, and insecurities enter the elderly person's life and interfere with any wisdom or ego integration that might have been possible. But for some, this can be a time of insightful reverie, integration, satisfaction, solace, and equanimity. It does not have to be a time of regret and despair.

Sequential Separations

There is another way to view the life cycle. It can be seen as a series of separations leading to various forms of healthy growth or to insecurity and isolation. Each period of separation may cause stress and harm to the individual or provide the opportunity for further maturation.

Separation begins with conception, at which time the fertilized egg separates into many cells, quickly differentiating into complex organs with a host of functions. The mystery remains as to how such a small group of cells differentiates to become the complete human being.

At the birth of the child, a violent separation occurs, and the infant is diverted from depending on the mother's blood for nourishment to depending on the mother's love and concern for feeding and caring. Before birth, the developmental process is more or less automatic, with varying degrees of success depending on heredity, nutrition of the mother, and prenatal care. After birth, there are numerous variables that affect the child's development, ranging from the ability of the mother to care for her child to the cultural differences that account for early training.

Another period of separation occurs when the child becomes mobile. Some parents move through this stage smoothly, others with fear and anxiety. While the child moves about and explores his or her environment, the parents may worry about the child being harmed in some way. It is a time that lays the groundwork for future abilities to separate easily from others. By contrast, it may be the beginning of many bouts of "separation anxiety." The child's reaction to separation and the parents' response to it will determine how subsequent separations will evolve.

The start of nursery school, day school, and baby-sitting are examples of the temporary but complete separation of the mother from the child for short and usually predictable amounts of time. These are times of stress for mother-child relationships, times when the child's confidence in the mother's ability to return is put to the test. Anxiety can increase when parents anticipate separation, which in turn can create doubt in the child. Pediatricians, child psychologists, and psychiatrists emphasize the importance of this time of separation. The same phenomenon occurs at the beginning of the formal school years, when there is a longer but predictable time of separation. It can be the start of an interesting relationship of the child with teachers and peers or, if the separation is poorly handled by parent and child, the beginning of a "school phobia." The child with this phobia either fears school or dreads separation from the security of home.

The next period of separation is more gradual and less dramatic. The child stays away from home for longer periods of time and occasionally wants to spend a night at a friend's house. If this stage progresses smoothly, more time is spent with peers and less time is spent at home. The child learns that home will still be there and is the base of operations. However, when the home is broken up by divorce or family tragedy, the wrenching separations can create considerable insecurity in the developing child.

With each change of school, from elementary to junior high and high school, there are more separations but there is also the chance to meet new friends and have new experiences. Many children have to adjust to their family's moving from one town, state, or country to another. With all of these changes, there is considerable stress, but there are also opportunities for new growth. Many children have the good fortune to spend weeks or months at summer camp. Although at times troublesome, this time away can lead to new growth for children as they reach far beyond their homes to develop a variety of new relationships.

The most obvious separation for young adults is the time when they leave home for their place in the adult world. When entering the workplace or attending college, young adults are still home based and dependent on their parent or parents. It is a time of great stress for some, whereas others seem to glide through this period with great equanimity. For some, the long-sought freedoms of the adult life are too overwhelming, and the responsibilities of the adult world are more than had been anticipated. We are now witnessing a new phenomenon: adult children are returning to the "empty nest" after years of living away from home.

When adults marry, the separation from home becomes more obvious and abrupt than at any other time—a new home, a new beginning, a new family, a repeat of the previous life cycle. Marriage is one of the tests of adulthood that involves compromise and accommodation as never before experienced by the participants. It is the test of separateness from parents and the simultaneous living together with another person with mutual benefits and responsibilities. During marriage, there are many separations that test the viability of the union. Later, with the birth of children into the family, the children themselves are engaged in their own separations and the parents are forced to relive the life cycle through them.

Throughout the ensuing years, each person experiences more separations. The moves from one place to another, the loss of friends, and the loss of former physical or mental abilities are other examples of separation issues that occur with aging.

Without a doubt, the most dramatic separation that adults must go through is the final separation that occurs with death. The deaths of parents, siblings, children, spouses, or friends all take their toll on the life of the survivor. Although death marks the end of the relationship as experienced in real life, the deceased person lives on in memory and the separation is never complete.

The ability to separate from others and the ability to stand alone when necessary are two of the central ingredients of adult life. As the life cycle goes on from one generation to another, the periods of separation are often the turning points in a person's life. Psychiatrists and other students of human behavior pay considerable attention to these times in child and adult development. It is important for the psychiatrist to be aware of the stage in the life cycle that corresponds to the patient's age. It is also important for the psychiatrist to determine whether the individual has successfully negotiated the various stages and attained the virtues and traits that are typical in these stages. When traumas to the developing ego have occurred, these must be noted. Such information can be useful in understanding and treating any prevailing disorders, whether these consist of symptoms, behavioral problems, or personality problems.

CHAPTER 3

HEREDITY, PARENTING, AND SOCIETY

Some years ago, when I first began to practice psychiatry, I encountered a mother who wanted to blame all of her son's bad behavior on one of the father's relatives. She was convinced that whatever he did, he was responding to traits that he inherited directly from his father's side of the family. She saw the resemblances on all occasions. I could not convince her that, perhaps, some of the behavior was caused by her misdirected parenting. At the time, it seemed to me that she was using heredity as a defense against her own inability to cope with her son's behavior. For example, when he failed to go to school or stayed out all night, she found it easy to explain: "His uncle did the same thing."

During the time that I was dealing with this family situation, I was still heavily influenced by the psychiatric thinking of the 1940s and 1950s, which stated, unequivocally, that the child's behavior was the direct result of parental influence. No quarter was given to hereditary factors at all. Such attitudes, which indicated that parents were responsible for the child's behavior, produced considerable guilt in parents when their children did not respond to parental guidance and discipline. The general line of thinking was, Is it any wonder those kids behave that way—just look at their parents. For many years, parents endured the accusations that they had caused their children's bad behavior. I remember speaking with a board member of a school for seriously disturbed children, who were suffering mostly from autism and childhood schizophrenia. His comment was, "It's no wonder that these children have problems. Just look at their parents." Here was an educated and altruistic man who was poorly informed on the developing trends, which pointed toward the bio-chemical and organic nature of these particular disorders.

In the intervening years, we have learned a lot about heredity and its influence on behavior. We have learned how some diseases are heavily tinged by heredity factors. We have learned about tempera-ment observed at birth and how such inborn temperament changes little in the developing child. The previously mentioned distressed mother was not entirely wrong in observing similar traits in family members, nor was I wrong in asserting that proper parenting was im-portant. Time has taught us that both child development and behav-ior are not so easily studied and understood. But there is another dimension to child rearing. Some time ago, I read that *children exert powerful influences in creating their environment.* I cannot remember where I first came upon this remark, but when I read it, I was struck with its basic truth. It reminded me of the fact that for years psychia-trists and other mental health workers have been assuming that par-ents, and to some extent society, were primarily responsible for the child's environment. But here was an observation that children also have a great effect in determining their own environment.

Although children are greatly influenced by their surroundings, most parents can attest to the fact that none of their children always react as expected to parental admonitions, directions, or discipline. Each child, in his or her own particular style, creates the world in which he or she lives in definitive ways. Although we are not always aware of it, we, as adults, also create to a large extent the world in which we live.

The developing child attends to and is alerted by the events and people in the environment that suit his or her basic nature. A passive child is attracted to quiet pursuits and is drawn to goals that require less energy. When interacting with people, he or she is more likely to go unnoticed and be easily swayed by the wishes of others. By contrast, an aggressive child will push his or her way through life, attending to his or her own wishes and desires. Often, the aggressive individual will ignore the needs of others around him or her. The basic temperament of a child will greatly influence how adults will interact with him or her.

In this chapter, I discuss the role of parenting, the impact of society on the developing child, and the recent research findings regarding heredity in mental illness.

A Look to the Past

Before the last century, the general population assumed that the behavior of children and adults was determined to a great degree by their hereditary background. It was really quite simple. Persons looked like their ancestors and they often acted like them. It was all self-evident. Of course, there were the old admonitions, such as "spare the rod and spoil the child," which indicated that parenting was of some importance. But when parenting went wrong, it was easy to blame a family member for the inherited traits. Then came the revolution that was to change the thinking of parents, educators, child and adult psychiatrists, and other psychotherapists. Heredity was no longer blamed for the behavior of the child. Parents became solely responsible for controlling and influencing their children's growth and development. No longer could they blame a child's behavior on inheritance from Father, Mother, Uncle Ned, or Cousin Anne.

It all began with a Viennese neurologist named Sigmund Freud. Although the father of psychoanalysis probably never intended it to turn out this way, children, parents, and the culture have not been the same since his discoveries.

Freud postulated that conflicts about sexuality and aggression were repressed—pushed into the unconscious—which in turn caused neurotic symptoms. The psychiatrist's task was to analyze the patient, uncover the conflicts, bring them to consciousness, and thus restore the patient to health.

The theory of the unconscious, the concept of defense mechanisms, analysis of dreams, and other "dynamic" issues originated by Freud form the foundation of psychotherapy to which most psychiatrists adhere in their work with neuroses. (For more information on this subject, see Chapter 7 in this volume.)

How do psychiatrists try to uncover the conflicts that confound patients? Patients who have recurrent neurotic depression, for example, usually repress their angry feelings. If the psychiatrist is able to bring to awareness the repressed anger in patients, he or she then can attempt to help the patients express this anger in an appropriate and effective manner. When this is successfully accomplished, patients can return to feeling well and free of depression. If patients learn the appropriate way to express their anger, they also will be able to prevent depression from recurring.

Child Rearing After Freud

The implication of the grand, imaginative scheme originated by Freud was that the child developed conflicts in early life because of poor or inadequate parenting. In contrast, if the parenting were proper and correct, the child would grow up with minimal conflicts and be free of neuroses.

Freud's theories thus formed the basis of psychoanalysis. His followers extrapolated much from what he said, perhaps far beyond what he intended, and this laid the groundwork for the massive parental guilt that has been evident in the ensuing years.

In Europe, and especially in the United States, psychoanalysts and others stated categorically or implied that child rearing had to be done in a loving way, free of the dogmatic and autocratic ways of Victorian parents. Later, in this country and abroad, changes evolved in educational institutions, with "open classrooms" where children were encouraged to express themselves and seek out their own level of work, free of teachers' demands or structure. In the offices of child therapists, the theme was permissiveness, allowance for the expression of feelings and understanding of the child's wishes. The child was to be encouraged and not thwarted in any way. (No doubt Freud would have objected to this distortion of his basic theories.) In the years that followed, a radical change had occurred from the strict discipline of the 19th and early 20th centuries to the permissiveness of the 1960s and 1970s.

Meanwhile, parents were convinced by authorities in child rearing that the child was born with a clean slate on which was engraved the imprint of the parents as they struggled with the question of how to properly raise their child. If the child turned out to be an educated citizen who married well and was successful in his or her vocational endeavors, the parents took the credit. If the child failed in any of these areas, it was the parents' fault. Nothing happened that was not controllable by parents or fixable by the child therapists. It all depended on reading the right books or talking to the correct authorities. Much of what was done in therapy with children and with adults involved guilt. What did the mother do to cause this outcome? Nothing happens to a child without a parent's causing it. Did anyone allow for the possibility of the existence of a "bad seed"? No self-respecting parent would allow for an outmoded idea such as the possibility of bad behavior coming from a hereditary base. Rather, it became fashionable to accept the blame like a good conscientious parent. There was enough guilt to spread around to everyone.

For parents so afflicted with guilt, long years of counseling by psychotherapists followed. And for the adult afflicted with neurotic symptoms, it took many long hours to figure out who represented the villain in the person's past. Having found the parent who was responsible for the neurotic adult, it remained the task of the analyst to repair the damage. This often took years. But finding out the cause of a particular neurotic behavior did not necessarily bring about a cure. Psychotherapists began to notice that it took more than an intellectual knowledge of one's past to manage a cure for neurotic symptoms. It took a motivated patient to change behavior and work through neurotic patterns.

Meanwhile, an interesting study was done on the subject of temperament. There were questions that often puzzled researchers. Was temperament inherited, did it change over years, and could it be modified by parental or societal influences? The basic findings in more than 140 healthy newborns who were studied for the next 20 years of their lives indicated that the temperament with which each child was born did not change significantly during the time from infancy to adulthood. (This study and its implications for child rearing are described in detail in Chapter 12 in this volume.)

Society As the Cause of Mental Illness

When I was in residency training in psychiatry in the late 1950s, a book called *Society As the Patient* had been published. The name intrigued me, as it touched on what I had observed to be an important influence in everyone's life. It was obvious that once a person was born, his or parents were of great significance to growth and development, but what about the impact of the media, of radio, television, and the printed page? Were not these factors also of great importance? If society had many flaws, was it not society as a whole that needed correction? Was it not society that really was the patient? Why were we putting all the blame on parents?

At that time, little was written about temperament or hereditary factors. The scientific literature and the lay press made few references to genetic determinants. It was the "age of the child"—sthe unrepressed child—and society did little to help the developing child repress his or her id impulses (basic biological impulses). Meanwhile, parents looked on as the child was influenced by the many inputs from his or her environment.

During the 20 years from the 1960s to the 1980s, many dramatic changes occurred. There never has been a period of greater social upheaval than during these two decades. Consider the many remarkable alterations in our society.

These were the two decades that saw the rise in drug abuse by the young, which killed many and injured large numbers both physically and psychologically. Simultaneously, the sexual revolution was born. It promised to allow free and uninhibited sexual expression with no physical or emotional cost. Unfortunately, there was a considerable price to pay for such unbridled sexual intimacy. One of the consequences was the breakdown of the nuclear family, which probably had been overidealized in the early part of the century. A second result was the increase in sex-linked diseases, the worst of which was acquired immunodeficiency syndrome (AIDS).

Meanwhile, the civil rights movement—long overdue—was born; women's liberation became a rallying point. Both brought about much unrest and stress in the general population. The rights of minorities and the rights of many groups not previously recognized, such as gay men and lesbians, were brought to the front page of newspapers. Authority figures were criticized, especially by the young, and everyone became an expert on political and social issues. Old religious and political groups were derided and demythologized. Anything old and venerable was considered irrelevant, and things "new" were given prominence. Of course, whatever was new did not remain so for long, as it was soon replaced by still another new object or idea. Planned obsolescence did not apply only to manufactured goods. Being older than age 30 was bad; being younger than 30 was "cool." Even in the field of mental health, there were psychiatrists in the United States, such as Thomas Szasz, who were saying that mental health was a myth. In England, R. D. Laing said that schizophrenic patients were simply reacting to society in ways that were appropriate, given the sickness that society displayed.

In the last few years still more rapid changes have occurred. Communism, the feared monster of previous decades, suddenly evaporated. In 1990, I attended a North Atlantic Treaty Organization (NATO) assembly meeting in Europe. For the first time in history, two men from opposing countries appeared on stage to express their views about the groups they led: General Galvin, of the United States, spoke on behalf of the NATO Alliance and General Ubov, of the Union of Soviet Socialist Republics, represented the Warsaw Pact. No one could have predicted, even 1 year before, that these two men would have made their appearances at the same meeting. The following year, the Soviet Union had virtually dissolved. Communism was dead, and some form of free enterprise was about to replace it.

The massive cultural movements that were evident in the 1960s and thereafter had a tremendous impact on the developing children who were exposed to these changes. The debasing of authority figures and institutions, the sexual freedoms, and the increased use of street drugs provided a powerful influence on the young. Meanwhile, another change was becoming more prevalent. The forces exerted by parents on their children were weakened, whereas the pressures of siblings and peers on the children were becoming more evident.

As society increasingly influenced the developing child, the effect of parents on children diminished. As parents became more powerless, they tended to blame the problems observed in their children on television, the school system, the government, and other factors. But while placing blame on societal factors, parents remained guilty for the outcome of their children; they had been conditioned for too many years to believe that they were solely responsible for their children's behavior.

Responses to Alterations in Society

When powerful institutions in society become less influential—when the family, the educational system, and religious institutions become less potent—there is a proliferation of new forces to fill the vacuum. The *commune* became the new family to which the young could escape. The Eastern guru replaced the preacher in the local church and the rabbi in the synagogue. Parents rushed to join self-help groups such as Tough Love, which tried to help parents deal with the aberrant behavior of their children. Individuals sought out sensitivity groups to help them to realize their potential for feeling the emotions that they had repressed. Others joined Erhard Seminars Training (EST) or LifeSpring, both of which discouraged blaming others for one's fate. These groups emphasized self-reliance and the acceptance of responsibility for the person's own life. Thus, in a secular way, many of these groups adhered to a basic principle contained in the Judeo-Christian heritage (i.e., each person is responsible for his or her own life and the life of others around him or her).

At present, another sweeping change is occurring. As more information is uncovered by researchers in the mental health field, it is becoming obvious that heredity is also important in the origin of some severe mental illnesses such as schizophrenia, bipolar disorder, and alcoholism. Heredity also may be of importance in some of the neurotic and behavioral disorders. Epidemiological studies and new techniques for viewing the brain have suggested that heredity may be more important in the development of mental and emotional illnesses than had been previously believed.

Heredity and Mental Illness

Research in the mental health field in the past has focused heavily on psychosocial issues that presumably have been responsible for various disorders. Urban crowding, poverty, fast-paced modern life, divorce, mobility of the population, and proper parenting have all been studied. Individual psychology and various social factors have been weighed to cull etiological factors contributing to mental illness.

More recently, mental health researchers have concentrated on hereditary factors. Research has yielded considerable new information particularly in the more serious mental illnesses, the psychoses. For example, there is now good evidence that schizophrenia and bipolar disorder have definite hereditary components. Only 20 years ago, the literature widely emphasized mothers who were cold and ineffective communicators; they were called "refrigerator parents" by researchers who studied them. These mothers were blamed for producing autistic and schizophrenic children. They also were referred to as "schizophrenogenic mothers." These parents, while engaged in child rearing, were said to give their children contradictory messages, thus creating a no-win situation for the children. The phenomenon was called a "double-bind" communication. For example, a mother may tell a child that she loves him or her and then embrace the child in a stiff and unaffectionate manner. The verbal and physical communication give opposite messages and leave the child confused. It is not difficult to imagine the guilt that such a parent experienced at the thought that he or she caused schizophrenic behavior in a child by inadequate and negligent parenting. All parents probably give double messages at some time to their children—without causing them to become schizophrenic. What parent has not said to an adolescent as he or she leaves the house for a date, "Have a good time but be very careful"?

Today, there is virtually no reference in psychiatric journals to such poor parenting of schizophrenic children. More evidence is accumulating that schizophrenia is biologically based, has a large hereditary component, and is not produced primarily by poor parenting. From the latest research findings, it is evident that schizophrenia is not caused by a single factor; it has many determinants. There are probably psychosocial factors that weigh heavily on individuals who are prone to schizophrenia, but the hereditary base needs to be present to produce the chemical changes in the brain found in schizophrenia. Most of the population would not become schizophrenic when exposed to profound stresses. But those unfortunate persons who have a strong hereditary predisposition toward the illness are likely to develop schizophrenia when subject to the same stress.

According to the National Institute of Mental Health (NIMH), research on schizophrenia has shown the following:

1. Approximately 1% of newborn children in this country will develop schizophrenia at some point in their lifetime.
2. Schizophrenia appears in every culture at about the same rate, 1%, referred to as the prevalence rate.
3. The rate of schizophrenia in siblings who are not twins is 10%–15%. That is, the brothers or sisters of schizophrenic individuals have a much higher rate of schizophrenia than the general population. However, if identical twins are raised by parents in separate households and one of the twins goes on to develop schizophrenia, the other is likely to become schizophrenic in about 40%–60% of cases. It is presumed that these statistics indicate evidence of a strong hereditary component.
4. When a child, without a family history of schizophrenia, is brought up by a schizophrenic parent, the child has no greater

chance of developing schizophrenia than does any other child in the same society.

5. In general, genetically close relatives are more likely to develop the illness. Distant relatives are thus much less subject to the disorder.

The aforementioned observations appear to be true for all countries that have been studied throughout the world, thus modifying the importance of cultural or family influences that might be responsible for schizophrenia. In contrast to what was believed only 50 years ago, schizophrenia is now viewed as being partially inherited. In addition, chemical abnormalities in the brain of schizophrenic patients have been uncovered; these can be altered by means of medication administered by psychiatrists. (More details about such medications can be found in Chapter 15 in this volume.)

Manic-depressive disorder is now called bipolar disorder in the new psychiatric classification in the fourth edition of the American Psychiatric Association's *Diagnostic and Statistical Manual of Mental Disorders*, or DSM-IV. Heredity is even more important in this illness than in schizophrenia. In bipolar disorder, there is a dominant gene that carries the illness from one generation to another. I frequently have seen patients with bipolar disorder who have a parent or other close relative who also has the disorder. In the past, patients with bipolar disorder often spent many months or years in psychiatric hospitals. Today, long hospital stays are unusual. With the discovery of the medication lithium, many of these patients' symptoms—their highs and lows—have been successfully controlled, and they have been able to work and carry out normal activities.

As reviewed in the seventh edition of *Kaplan and Sadock's Synopsis of Psychiatry*, studies on families who have bipolar disorder show an amazingly high percentage of the illness in relatives. In identical twins, if one twin contracts the disorder, there is a 33%–90% chance that the other twin will eventually become ill with bipolar disorder. The term for this phenomenon is *concordance*. The same statistic occurs even if the twins are raised separately. The concordance rate in nonidentical or fraternal twins is about 19%. Thus, heredity plays a large part in the origin of the illness, necessitating appropriate genetic counseling for young persons who have a family history of the disorder.

In the anxiety disorders, there are fewer research data on the hereditary influences. Some traits seem to run in families. For example, obsessional traits such as cleanliness and orderliness may be seen in family members. Nervousness and a tendency to worry also are common in families. But there is no real evidence that these traits are inherited. It is quite likely that children acquire these traits through their environments.

Statistics from NIMH summary reports indicate that one of the anxiety disorders, panic disorder, may be partially inherited. Studies on identical twins with panic disorder show that if one twin has the illness, there is a 31% chance (concordance) the other also will get the disorder. In fraternal twins, there is 0% concordance for this disorder. But this is the only anxiety disorder that shows such a concordance in identical twins.

There is now much evidence that alcoholism is inherited to some degree. According to NIMH summary reports, research has demonstrated that if one parent is alcoholic, there is a 25% chance that the offspring will be alcoholic. If both parents are alcoholic, the rate rises significantly to 50%. It is quite unlikely that alcoholism among the offspring would be due only to environmental factors. When the children of alcoholic parents observe in their parents inconsistent and poor behavior, one would expect considerable negative reinforcement for the drinking behavior. It would seem unlikely that the children would then mimic such behavior if there were not another strong compulsion to do so. Presumably, the compulsion to drink is due to hereditary factors.

Furthermore, studies with identical twins show that if one twin becomes alcoholic, the other has a 25% chance of doing the same. In the case of fraternal twins, the figure drops to 12%, which is about twice the rate of the general public. These NIMH statistics would indicate that there is a significant hereditary component in alcoholism.

As more information is uncovered through research on heredity and psychiatric illnesses, it will become possible to provide genetic counseling to couples who are anticipating having children. For example, if a young woman has bipolar disorder and plans to marry, she and her husband should know the statistical probabilities of their offspring getting the disorder. I have had occasion to do such counseling with young couples. If they have children and symptoms develop later in their children's lives, it would be beneficial for parents to have foreknowledge of this possibility so that early treatment could be obtained.

Genetic research also involves the attempt to locate specific genes on chromosomes in the cells of patients with psychiatric illnesses, especially the major psychoses, schizophrenia, and bipolar disorder. Attempts are being made to do the same in patients with Alzheimer's disease, diabetes, Huntington's chorea, and Down's syndrome.

In research with animals, it even has been possible to split certain genes and then recombine them to eliminate an undesirable illness. This research actually was done with the so-called shiverer mouse. These animals have a genetic abnormality: they lack the covering on nerve fibers necessary for the transmission of nerve impulses. This feature causes them to have a tremor that cannot be voluntarily controlled. Researchers have taken the affected genes, split and recombined them, and injected them into the bone marrow of the affected mouse. By so doing, the mouse has been "cured" of its shivering. It develops normal nerve fibers and is restored to health.

Researchers eventually will be able to do the same with humans. Split and recombined genes will be placed into the embryo, bone marrow, or central nervous system of affected persons with genetic disorders in the hope that the disorder will be eliminated.

As time goes on, much more will be discovered through research in the mental health field. Such research is in its early stages, and new and exciting developments can be expected in the coming years.

Conclusion

What factors are most responsible for the development of mental illness? Is genetic endowment more important than parenting? Are the influences that the child experiences from today's media of more significance than genetics or proper parenting? The answers to these questions are not completely available to us at this time. There is little doubt that all the factors mentioned are important.

In the disorders defined as psychoses, genetic factors appear to be of greater significance than psychiatrists had previously thought. Schizophrenia and bipolar disorder certainly have genetic foundations. In the neuroses, genetic factors do not seem certain, although more evidence is accruing in this direction. Organic illnesses, such as alcoholism, also show heavy genetic loading. Even the temperament of the newborn child, which changes little with growth and development, has been shown to be important in determining the child's reaction to various life stresses.

With all the genetic evidence available, how important is parenting? Few mental health workers would deny that effective parenting skills contribute to healthy child development. But the best parenting skills do not necessarily guarantee a successful outcome in child rearing. It depends heavily on the mixture of various personalities of parents and their children. Some parents handle aggressive children very well; others do so poorly. There are parents who cannot stand quiet children; others prefer them.

It is remarkable that some children will grow up with intact personalities and relatively free from psychiatric illness, even with the most horrendous family backgrounds. These are the survivors, the children who seem to have an inner strength that is probably genetic in origin. It allows them to cope with almost any circumstance and still come out ahead emotionally.

The influence of the culture is hard to measure. Intuitively, many individuals feel that the media have a large impact on today's children. Who can doubt the negative effect of violence on television? Does the constant visualization of violence make one inured to such acts? It may be difficult to prove, but it is quite likely that our media are having a profound influence on our children. What attitudes are being promulgated? What values are being expressed? What messages are being received? Researchers and psychotherapists in the mental health field should be speaking up about these influences, but parents, on their own, also should be exercising their judgments on these matters.

As time goes on, the various factors involved in producing psychiatric illnesses will become clearer. Researchers are working diligently toward deciphering the essential basis for these debilitating illnesses.

CHAPTER 4

STRESS AND COMMON EMOTIONAL REACTIONS

Everybody complains about stress, and most individuals think of their stress as the worst kind. A businessman tells me that his stress is unbelievable in the present economic environment, with the competition that exists and the sluggish spending of his customers. A homemaker says that some days her stress is beyond what anyone should bear, with sick and emotionally upset children and a husband with job problems. A physician complains that there is no one who has the stress that he encounters with emergency surgery, unhappy patients, malpractice worries, and the government on his back about Medicare.

Everyone complains about stress. Animal lovers even worry about stress on their pets. There are now counselors available for pet owners and their pets. Recently, I read about the effect of music on cows; while hearing a certain ballad, cows produced about 35% more milk than they did without the music. It seems every creature is under stress.

People have asked me how I can stand the stress of listening to the emotional and psychological problems of patients hour after hour. In contrast, I have a difficult time understanding how anyone can stand the stress of being a police officer, a fire fighter, an airline pilot, or a chief executive officer of a large company or the challenge of being a money manager, who handles billions of dollars of other people's money every day. I would rather be a psychiatrist! But I suppose it is not that stressful or complicated to do any one of the foregoing jobs, if you have a natural inclination toward the work and have been properly trained in the various fields.

Although stress appears to be a companion for all of us, it is not well understood. What really is stress? Borrowing a definition from physics, stress is a force or physical energy exerted on objects or bodies. When we are stressed, our bodies are required to respond in order to adjust to the stress. There is an attempt on the part of the body to bring the situation back to its former state. Some years ago, a researcher named Cannon called this phenomenon "homeostasis." He said that when a body is stressed in whatever manner, it tended, following the stress, to always return to its former state of equilibrium.

The originator of the modern concept of stress is the researcher and physiologist Hans Selye. In *Stress Without Distress*, Selye defines stress as "the non-specific response of the body to any demand made upon it" (p. 14). He developed the theory that the body adapted to stress by means of the endocrine system. He discovered that any perceived stress impacts an individual's brain and affects the hypothalamus, which in turn stimulates the pituitary gland. This organ, often referred to as the master gland or controlling gland of the endocrine system, then sends messages via hormones to other glands. These hormones stimulate the thyroid, parathyroid, adrenal glands, and sexual organs (testes and ovaries). Under stress, the thyroid gland can become more active, and the adrenal glands can produce an appropriate amount or an excess of adrenaline, cortisone, and related hormones. In this manner, as well as in other minute ways, the body is provided with the hormones that are required to meet a challenge and deal with the ensuing stress.

When the challenge requires a physical response, the body works efficiently to increase the blood supply to the large muscles, increase the heart and respiratory rate, dilate the pupils, and simultaneously slow down other organs, such as the digestive system. The individual organism therefore is able to handle emergencies or any stressful activity that may be consciously chosen, such as an athletic contest. When the requirement is a physical response, it is relatively automatic and consists of a primitive biological reaction.

When the response called for is of a psychological nature, the reaction is more complicated. In such cases, the autonomic nervous system plays an important role. If the nerves controlling the intestines, bladder, heart, lungs, and other systems are not properly regulated, diseases in these various organs may occur. Illnesses such as stomach or duodenal ulcers, colitis, asthma, cardiac arrhythmias, and neurodermatitis are possible results. Such diseases do not come about if the stress is momentary or happens only occasionally. They are more likely to be found if the stress is frequent and of long duration.

Fear, Anxiety, and Panic

When a sudden stress occurs, the various hormonal and organ systems in the body react in what has been referred to by Selye as a "fight or flight reaction." That is, individuals are prepared to enter into a fight to preserve their integrity or save their lives, or they are equipped to escape the perceived danger by running away. If the stimulus that provokes such a reaction is seen to be clearly dangerous or life threatening, the response of most people is one of fear. For example, if someone confronts another person and suddenly points a gun at that person's head, the appropriate reaction is *fear*. In contrast to the fear response, *anxiety* is an expectation of something bad happening to the individual. The anxiety may concern an event about to occur, such as an examination or the anticipation of confronting a common phobia. Or the anxiety may have no fixed focus and is then referred to as a free-floating anxiety. The state of *panic*, on the other hand, differs from both anxiety and fear in that there is usually no stimulus at all that is responsible for the reaction. Panic comes on suddenly, appears to be unprovoked, and has a more profound effect on the individual. When experiencing a panic disorder, individuals are so distraught that they feel they are going to faint, lose their minds, or simply die. A panic disorder is more difficult to endure than acute anxiety or a known phobia. Some patients even attempt suicide rather than face more panic attacks.

Is All Stress Bad?

Everyone has been stressed in favorable ways. When we experience a joyful moment, it is a type of stress. However, it usually has favorable physiological effects on our bodies. Norman Cousins, in his book *Anatomy of an Illness*, suggested laughter as a positive stress toward the attainment of health. When I stress myself at tennis or skiing, I am enjoying this form of stress on my body and mind, which is a pleasant physical activity that I presume will be helpful to my well-being. Even the stress of giving a speech to a large audience can result in positive feelings, which in the long run may be mentally healthy. Mild stress that is felt to be emotionally congruent with goals or aspirations can result in positive feelings, whether this stress is in sports, family life, or business. It is a mistake to try to avoid all stress. By doing so, many persons live a life with little enjoyment—a life that is lived defensively with few moments of genuine pleasure.

Whether one feels a certain activity as stressful depends on the person. Although some individuals anticipate skiing down a steep, bumpy trail as an exhilarating and positive stress, others would consider it a frightening experience to be avoided at all cost. Rock climbing looks dangerous and perhaps a bit extreme to most of us, but to some devotees of this sport, it is a stimulating and enjoyable stress. I know military men who are experienced paratroopers. When they feel stressed by their day-to-day work in the office, they call the local base where parachute jumping is available, they schedule a jump or two, and after completing their jumps, they find that their tension is considerably relieved.

There are stresses that most people would agree are unpleasant, but there is no stress that is universally difficult for everyone. This fact becomes obvious when one looks at the common stresses listed in magazine articles on stress. The death of a loved one and the loss of a job are considered among the highest forms of stress on these lists. Other stresses such as traveling and changing positions at work are less stressful to most individuals. But even in this rating of stress levels, there is a vast difference between what two individuals regard as major stress. For example, in a marriage that is fraught with problems and where the couple is on the verge of divorce, the death of one of the partners may not be regarded as extremely stressful. It is conceivable that death of the spouse could be experienced by the survivor as a relief. To some individuals, moving from one job to another represents a stimulating opportunity, while to others it is a frightening and upsetting experience. The perception of stress is, like the appreciation of art, in the eye of the beholder.

Stress and the Modern Age

Has stress really increased in modern times? It is my opinion that stress is greater now than in the past. Consider what has happened in the last 200 years. Society has moved from an agricultural base, with light industry such as shipbuilding, glassblowing, home building, and weaving, to an industrial society. Most of the former activities were done by hand with the use of simple tools. All articles of clothing were made by hand at home or by the local tailor. One could not go to a clothing store and purchase a suit or coat. It had to be made to order and fitted to the particular person's needs and requirements. Today, most clothing is manufactured by the large industries designed to make articles in all sizes and shapes to fit individual needs.

For everyone, life in the 1700s was very physical. Almost everyone was physically stressed to work many hours of every day. Most people living at that time were likely to get enough exercise to satisfy their cardiovascular requirements. There was little time for leisure. And it is quite likely that much of the stress of everyday life was drained off by the enormous amount of physical work that was required just to survive. Pumping water from the well, growing fruits and vegetables, caring for animals, and traveling via horseback or carriage all required much physical exertion.

Today, life is physically much simpler. With the advent of modern industry, the need to make objects by hand was largely replaced by mass production. The automobile has made us all physically weaker than our ancestors, unless we make special efforts to walk, jog, swim, or find some other recreation to satisfy our needs for physical exertion. In modern times, our bodies are required to deal with stressors that are much more emotional in nature than physical. Most of our problems and anxieties require a mental solution rather than a physical assault. However, our anatomical makeup, our endocrine system, and the way in which our bodies respond to stress have remained the same, whereas the satisfaction of our needs has changed considerably from past centuries. Because most of our stressors are not physical in origin but mental, and because we physically do not work off these stresses as well as our ancestors did in the past, it is my belief that we are consciously aware of more stress now than ever before.

Other Societal Changes

There are a number of other stressors in our society that are integral to modern life. Before the invention of the automobile, train, and airplane, people traveled little from their place of birth. Traveling was difficult, costly, and risky. Furthermore, there was little need to go beyond one's hometown. Only the adventurous took long journeys or sailed to other lands. Most people did not travel more than a short distance from their homes. Today, it is not unusual for the modern businessperson or executive to fly to various parts of the world each year, change jobs, and relocate many times in the course of his or her career. It is estimated that about one-fourth of the population move to a different address each year. Such frequent moves are quite stressful to the families involved.

Consider also how frequently we are expected to change the clothing styles that we wear, the cars that we drive, and the playthings that are so quickly outmoded, even the computers that we own. Everything that we possess is old before its usefulness is outdated. We are bombarded by advertising that suggests a built-in obsolescence. Built-in obsolescence is a new phenomenon that is unique to our civilization. Never before have there been so many choices, so many options, and so many ways to be dissatisfied with our current possessions, experiences, or goals. Through the subtlety of the constant barrage of advertising, we are assaulted by needs that we never knew we had. Our physical and psychological needs are exploited daily with incessant reminders that life could be better, if only we possessed yet one more new object, traveled to one more different place, or won the lottery. Our children grow up thinking that the whole world has more than they do. It is striking that despite all of our physical comforts, adequate nutrition, and possibilities for living well, so many of us are unhappy with our lives.

Today, the youth of our nation are overly programmed in the early years in preschool, day care, elementary school, town athletic programs, and dance, music, or art classes. Then, beginning in high school and especially in college, adolescents are on their own with little support. At that time, they are given unlimited freedom in a world for which they are not prepared. There are few rules for social behavior. At colleges, the administrators, having been intimidated by the uprisings of the 1960s and 1970s, have all but given up their supervision of college students. In my role as a psychiatric consultant to colleges, I have been amazed at the degree of alcohol abuse, drug use, and sexual permissiveness that have become the norm on campus. Interpersonal relationships and mutual commitments have reached a new low. All this has created more stress on the young people of today.

Meanwhile, our institutions have become demythologized to such an extent that the young have little regard or appreciation for the founding, growth, or importance of our political, religious, or educational institutions. Perhaps this lack of appreciation has always been true of the young, who often have sought new ideas and views on everything. To many of them, nothing is useful or important unless it is new and current. Anything old is not revered. This attitude leads to a lack of institutional continuity, which has created in society an anxiety for the young that has not been present in past generations.

No previous century has experienced the rapid changes that we now observe. Much of this change is due to our ability to communicate on such a broad level through television, radio, newspapers, and magazines. The Internet and on-line computer services contribute even more information to absorb. Whereas newspapers have the "latest" editions, the TV newscasters and politicians work on their 10-second sound bites. News becomes old almost as soon as it is heard or read. In addition, every tragedy, such as fires, murders, and suicides, is graphically displayed on the news. More recently, *Prime Time*, *Hard Copy*, and other TV programs that supposedly provide the inside story of events have left TV viewers more cynical than ever about institutions, politicians, and people in power. All of these changes are confusing to the general public, and they certainly add to our general level of stress.

Stress in the Developing Child

There are various factors that contribute to stress as the child develops from infancy into adulthood. There is little doubt that physical stressors in the pregnant mother have an effect on the growing fetus; there is direct evidence of physical effects. For example, if the pregnant mother consumes too much alcohol, it is quite likely that a fetal alcohol syndrome may result. In this syndrome, there is retardation of growth in both height and weight. Malformation of the skull, brain, and heart, as well as other abnormalities, may occur. This syndrome is completely preventable by the mother's abstinence from alcohol during pregnancy. Similarly, if the mother's hormones that flow to the fetus via the umbilical cord either are in excess or are deficient, certain abnormalities will result. The hormones from the pituitary, thyroid, adrenal, and sex glands all affect the growing fetus profoundly. Viral infections and protein deficiencies are also of great importance. Such effects are known and are observable.

Although emotional stress on the mother probably plays a large part in the well-being of the fetus, the specific effects of this type of stress during pregnancy are not known and have not been measured. The same can be said of birth. Aside from physical injuries at birth, there is no documented evidence that birth, in itself, causes any great psychological injury to the infant, despite psychoanalytical theories referred to as "birth trauma" and "primal scream."

Although the possible emotional stressors on the growing fetus are not known, it has become evident that what happens to the infant immediately after birth is extremely important to normal growth and development. Satisfied and secure parents certainly are going to create a greater feeling of comfort and security in the infant than are hostile, feuding parents. A calm, nurturing mother will do a better job of mothering than a hysterical, detached, or uncertain person.

There are a number of common stressors that impinge on the developing child. (For further details on how children grow and develop, see Chapter 2 in this volume.)

At first, the infant becomes attached to the mothering one, who meets the child's physical and emotional needs. This attachment is referred to as bonding. Any prolonged interruption in providing these needs causes stress in the infant. As this bonding and attachment grows and the infant becomes aware of his or her mother, a social smile develops at about age 2 months. Although an interest in others subsequently develops, the infant also begins to fear strangers. How the parents handle these various stages is of significance, since overreacting to any stage may cause undue stress to the growing infant. For example, it has been demonstrated that anxiety in the parents is keenly felt by the infant, and the resulting stress is manifested by reactions such as poor eating or frequent crying.

Another stressor for the growing child is separation from the parents. A certain degree of separation anxiety is normal for infants, but some develop undue anxiety from these experiences. If parents are too concerned about leaving the infant, this alone creates anxiety. If not handled properly during the development of the child, separation anxiety may continue into childhood as a school phobia and into adult life as a neurotic condition such as agoraphobia (i.e., fear of being away from the security of home).

Recently, there has been increasing concern about sexual and physical abuse that has occurred in childhood. It has become evident that there has been more abuse of all kinds than had been realized by the experts in the past. There is little doubt that abuse is stressful and often leads to great psychological pain. Although there is the danger of parents and clinicians overreacting to this phenomenon, it is necessary to recognize that much abuse exists. At this point, little is known about the psychological causes of abuse, but certain conditions provide a breeding ground for abuse. Alcohol and substance abuse by parents or other caregivers no doubt contributes to physical and sexual abuse. It has been documented that abused children often grow up to become abusive adults, thus continuing the cycle. In addition, abusive behavior is found in persons with certain personality disorders, mental disorders such as schizophrenia, and abnormalities in sexual desire (paraphilias).

Perhaps one of greatest stressors in childhood is the failure to be accepted by a peer group. Children severely feel the effects of isolation and rejection by their peers. Many children, and particularly adolescents, compromise their integrity for the sake of a sought-after group identity. Under the influence of the group, many youngsters will do things that they would be incapable of doing alone. Although being part of a group is important, the individual also must seek an identity of his or her own. Adolescents often try on one "mask" after another until they find an identity that suits them. This process usually takes years. Meanwhile, much stress is encountered along the way.

The absent or uninvolved parent is another common stressor for the developing child. Because of the increase in divorce, the single-parent household is becoming more prevalent. Many more children now will spend some of their childhood years living in single-parent households. Introducing stepparents into the family also adds to the stress. Although these changes do not always result in more stress, the potential for additional stress is present in these homes.

Many children are faced with the failure to learn skills appropriate for their age. In school, these skills may involve reading, writing, and arithmetic or mastering other basic skills needed to take a responsible place in society. At the same time, athletic and social skills also must be learned. Failure to acquire a certain degree of success in these skills often leads to low self-esteem and feelings of failure, symptoms of physical distress, or depression.

Despite all the difficulties to overcome, most children manage to succeed well enough to attain a satisfactory place in their world.

When they reach adolescence, the stresses become even greater. At puberty, the hormonal changes that occur demand new adjustments for both sexes. Adolescence seems to take longer as we have become more civilized. A century ago, a child became a working contributor to society at about age 12 or 14 years. Now, many children are biological adults, age 20 or 25, before they leave the protective surroundings of their home to seek their own fortunes. More recently, we are witnessing the return of the young to their parental homes after age 25, 30, or even 35 and older, with or without their own children. Returning to the homes of their parents produces stress for the parents as well as the adult children.

The stress of sexual identity and relationships with peers, along with the choice of companion or mate, is among the biggest hurdles for the teenager to overcome. Researchers tell us that the sexual identity of a person is determined early, at about age 3 years or younger. If this is true, developing individuals have no choice but to adjust to what they feel to be their natural inclination as they grow older. If a male child feels that he is more female than male in his identity leanings, he may have no choice but to become homosexual. This discovery is startling compared to our former concepts of the development of sexual identity (i.e., that the sexual identity of children depends on the parenting to which they are exposed in family life). For example, it was believed that a domineering mother and a passive father could produce a homosexual son. There is little evidence that this actually happens. The stress on children who feel homosexually driven must be enormous, even with the relative acceptance of the gay community today. Of course, these sexual identities are not always so clear. The result is that some individuals grow up experimenting with one sexual orientation or the other; behaviorally, they may be bisexual.

But even for those who develop the expected male or female identities, the struggle for acceptance by peers or by a significant other presents its own stresses. Many a lover has fallen into a profound depression over the loneliness and lowered self-esteem that followed a rejection by his or her mate. The stress during this period may be continuous or intermittent, but it is without doubt a turbulent time for many young people.

As important as sexual identity is in the life of the growing person, it also is essential that he or she identifies with significant role models. Parents, relatives, and teachers play a large part in this identity. Most successful persons with whom I have spoken attribute their identification with such role models as a major factor in giving their lives direction and inspiration toward a specific goal. I know a high school teacher who was directly responsible for a number of students going to college, many of whom would have failed to do so had it not been for the inspiration of this competent teacher. By his stimulating manner and teaching skills, he prodded his students to pursue a wide variety of academic courses.

Little is known about why a child identifies with one adult and not another. Furthermore, we do not know exactly why a child identifies with one of his or her peers as opposed to another. It makes a big difference whether a child identifies with a disturbed teenager who acts out or an honor student who has goals and direction. Often the child takes his or her identity from many of those in his or her environment. An identity with a cultural hero such as a rock star or sports figure may last for years. Usually, such idols are replaced by other cultural heroes as the child grows older.

Later, as adults, many individuals take on somewhat older persons as mentors with whom to identify. This mentoring occurs in young adult life, when individuals reach their 20s and 30s, and often occurs in the vocational setting, although it can be seen in social and interpersonal settings as well. By the time middle age arrives, most of this type of identification is complete.

Adult Stress

The major stressors in adult life concern vocation, interpersonal relationships, health, and financial security. To some individuals, job stress is the most significant concern; to others, marriage is the biggest concern. Others are preoccupied with financial aspirations and worry about their failure to attain sufficient monetary security.

Vocational stresses are many. They vary from the tedious routine work that many persons experience to the high-tech life-or-death decisions of the surgeon, from the day-to-day concerns of the mother with her children to the high-risk stakes of the investment banker or the inner-city police officer on the beat. The stress that each person encounters differs with each job. However, it seems to me that the perceived stress of a job is highly individual to each person. I have known many individuals who can manage their jobs with minimal stress until a significant change occurs in the workplace. For example, engineers may function well in assignments related to their technical abilities, but as they progress in their jobs, they may be promoted to a managerial level and asked to write proposals, for which the engineers are not suited. Some may be expert technicians but not trained planners or administrators. I have known other professionals who have been under considerable stress because of their discomfort with new work assignments. Conversely, with other job changes, many persons feel much less stress in their new roles.

Various alterations in the workplace or in personnel can result in job stress. A new boss, new owners in a company takeover, downsizing of the work force for the financial benefit of the company, rapid growth of a small company, and changes in economic conditions all can result in new or additional stress for employees. With the recession during the late 1980s and early 1990s, many workers became unemployed. In addition, many employees were asked to retire prematurely. Such unemployment, for whatever reasons, usually causes enormous stress in those affected.

While consulting with patients in my office, I often have been asked questions relating to work stresses. The most common question is, Should I change my job? I do not think that I, as a psychiatrist, should engage in the business of advising individuals to change jobs, buy houses, get married, or make other important decisions. Rather, my role is to help patients clearly understand what conflicts they have with their choices and help them work out their own decisions regarding alternatives. If a patient chooses to leave his or her job after thoroughly understanding the issues involved, then it is his or her decision and responsibility to do so. Often, after reflecting on the job problems and figuring out the basic sources of stress, a patient alters his or her behavior and thinking, resulting in far less stress. He or she

then may keep that job. At times, however, the person has no alternative but to leave the stressful situation and relocate. The psychiatrist's job is to help define the problem rather than to determine
choices.

Interpersonal stressors come in all varieties and situations. A new
marriage, job, or friendship may bring on interpersonal stress that
was not present previously. Interpersonal stressors may involve
feelings of being put down, embarrassed, rejected, or forgotten by
others.

The security that most of us seek is obtained by the relationships
we have with others. An American psychiatrist, Harry Stack Sullivan, once stated that anxiety in humans is brought about most often
by the perceived approval or disapproval of significant others. It was
his opinion that nothing caused anxiety in a person more than his or
her concern with acceptance by others. Sullivan's theory is certainly
true for many people, although it does not seem to be so for all. There
are some individuals with personality disorders, such as those with
narcissistic and antisocial personality disorders, who do not appear to
be at all concerned with what others think of them nor do they suffer
from anxiety. But for most of us, the perceived evaluation of our
friends, relatives, co-workers, and acquaintances does mean a great
deal to our self-evaluation—to our self-esteem. Most of us have
a need for someone to feel deeply about us, to feel close, and to know
that person will be available to meet both our emotional and physical
needs.

Health issues are an obvious concern to most of us. Some individuals appear abnormally preoccupied with health, whereas others
pay little attention to their physical well-being. In the United States,
we are probably overly concerned with our health. A few years ago,
while on a tour of the health care system in Canada, I heard an important Canadian physician refer to Americans as "health care junkies."
Nowhere in the Western world do people go to physicians as much as
they do in the United States. We do have the most sophisticated
health care system in existence, but we are not necessarily the
healthiest civilization on the globe. Worry and concern about health
matters cause some to seek the help of physicians all too often. Others with hypochondriasis are determined to find the serious but elu-

sive disease that they feel exists. Still others obsessively obtain one consultation after another to determine exactly what disease they have. Billions of dollars are spent each year on the health care system, on over-the-counter remedies, and on quack cures that have not been scientifically tested. Health care issues represent a huge industry.

I have encountered patients who seem overly concerned with their health and who consume excessive amounts of vitamins and health foods, not just with the desire to live a healthy life but with the hope or even the expectation to live forever. When a disease strikes, they search in vain for what they did wrong, believing they did not supply the correct ingredient in their diet. It is as though they would like complete control of their lives, and they fully expect to be symptom and disease free. Although such a goal cannot be attained, billions of dollars are spent because of the hope that perfect health is achievable.

Financial security probably is on the top of the list of concerns for most people. Most individuals do not aspire to become enormously wealthy, but most do want to be financially secure. Feeling financially secure is especially evident among the elderly, who, despite adequate savings and obvious security, frequently complain bitterly about the cost of living and how things used to be. When asked if they have enough money, they admit readily that they have sufficient funds, but their insecurity about finances persists.

Among young people, the concern about money is more immediate. They want to know how to obtain more for getting that new car or stereo—now. But young adults also worry about their future security. The old American dream, home ownership for everyone and a level of financial security that goes beyond that of one's parents, is beginning to fade. Even white-collar workers, whose jobs were secure in the past, no longer have the same guarantee that they will be employed without interruption. At present, the leaders of industry are not certain of their future either. Whole companies are bought and sold and top officials are discharged. Many do not obtain new positions readily, thus causing tremendous stress for those unfortunate enough to be caught in this situation.

On the other hand, an enormous number of people play the lottery every day or gamble away their meager savings in the hope of making a big win. It is especially sad to see senior citizens who are not wealthy gamble away their money at the casinos, thus creating more insecurity and stress for themselves. In almost all cultures, the wealthy are revered even if they obtained the money illegally. Wealth symbolizes power, and the wealthy are seen as having power to do almost anything.

For many people, the lack of financial security is a tremendous stress. Few can feel secure without at least some financial base. But there also are many individuals who worry about money excessively, even though they have enough to support 10 families. It appears to me that financial security is relevant to what an individual wishes to achieve and what he or she has had. Most of us have heard stories of the Great Depression of the 1930s, such as the story of the wealthy man who had $10 million and lost $9 million in the stock market. He felt so depressed that he jumped out of a window, despite the fact that his remaining $1 million was more than what 99% of the population possessed.

There also are individuals who are never satisfied with what they have and are constantly working hard at obtaining even more. The motion picture *Wall Street* portrayed this effort to obtain more wealth well. It was clear that greed was the motivating factor in the lives of the characters in the movie. The attainment of money is stressful to both the greedy and the victims of greed.

Love may make the world go 'round, but money appears to be a driving force at least equal to love. Money also has been implicated as the root of all evil. Much of the stress of everyday life results from how a person perceives his or her financial security, whether the actual money he or she possesses is adequate or not. There are many individuals who have little of the world's goods to call their own but who have enormous emotional and spiritual security. These people do not long to win the lottery or make it big in Atlantic City.

Stress in adult life can arise from many sources. The general topics I have discussed in this chapter cover most of these sources. However, the origins of stress are unique to the individual, such as the loss of a loved one, the loss of health with the sudden onset of illness, and other losses that have private meaning to someone. These losses are not easily categorized. *Illness* for one person does not mean the same for another. The loss of financial security to some means little, whereas to others it is catastrophic. Everybody has their vulnerabilities—their own Achilles' heel—with which they must deal as best as they can. Everybody deals with stress in remarkably different ways. In the next chapter, I discuss the various ways of thinking about stress and managing stress.

CHAPTER 5

MANAGING STRESS

Most of us want to get rid of stress as soon as we encounter it. It's a lot like pain. We say, "Let's not talk about it. I just want to get relief." In our culture, there is little tendency to try to figure out what we may be doing to bring about stress or how we could avoid it. But these are important considerations.

There are several important questions we should ask ourselves when we encounter stress. The first is, What have I been doing to bring on stress? Too often, we are tuned in to how others cause us stress: "If it wasn't for my awful boss, I wouldn't have this stress" or "With a husband like that, who wouldn't have stress?" In our own defense, we usually blame those around us for making life difficult. And many times, difficult people do cause us stress. But it is useful to look at our own actions to see if stress could be avoided. Maybe there are things that we do or say that bring on bad reactions from those with whom we come in contact.

Case Example

A married woman came to see me about a problem with her husband. She complained that her husband frequently came home in the evening in a bad mood and got upset with her. She saw no reason why this should happen, as she had done nothing to provoke such behavior from him. Although he had some conflicts at work, he seemed to handle them well enough, although it left him tense when he arrived home. This tension caused his wife great stress.

In discussing the typical scene in her home upon her husband's arrival, she said that she usually rejected his anger and hostility toward her and defended herself by saying that he should not become angry at her for things that happen at the office. Of course, she was right technically. But what her husband needed was not a defensive reaction by her but some understanding of his emotional needs. I suggested to my patient that although she was not to blame for her husband's job problems, it would be wise to accept his irritable mood and postpone any reaction to it until after dinner. She followed this advice, and frequently his mood changed and he was quite cordial after dinner. On occasion, he even apologized for being so nasty when he came home. Eventually, he was able to modify his reactions and postpone expression of his feelings until a more suitable time. By his doing so, the stress on both husband and wife was decreased.

Another way of looking at stress is to focus on its purpose. This statement may seem absurd; after all, most of us want to get rid of stress. We don't want to think about stress having a purpose. However, the stress that we feel may be an important signal. Our bodies may be telling us to slow down, reassess what we are doing, think about our actions, or look again at our reasons for a particular behavior. *Few situations become stressful until our minds make them so.* The following case example illustrates this point.

Case Example

Some time ago, I spoke with a young man in his 30s, who had been married for several years. He had been sexually active before his marriage and had never had any problems with impotency. In fact, he was proud of his ability to become easily aroused, and his sexual relationship with his wife was quite satisfactory. However, he had recently become emotionally involved with another woman. Upon attempting a sexual liaison with this woman, he was completely impotent. His impotence caused him much stress, and he requested treatment.

Reflecting on his situation, I wondered what his body was telling him about his behavior. I told him to consider this question and think about his involvement with the second woman. It did not take him long to figure out that in his mind he was having sexual thoughts, but his body was not cooperating. After some discussion, it became clear that this man was not able to detach himself from his marriage and engage in an affair. Nor did he really want to be disloyal and deceptive to his wife. He quickly discontinued his new relationship, and his stress disappeared.

Although stress cannot always teach us something about ourselves, it is worth looking at our stress to see if we are doing things that are not necessary or are really harmful to our well-being.

Should we try to get rid of all stress? Not only is it impossible to do, but also it is undesirable. A certain degree of stress keeps us alert and on top of things. A mild amount of stress prepares us for the competitive world in which we live. But too much stress gets in our way. It prevents us from performing at our best.

Basic Needs for Good Mental Health

Patients and caregivers alike need to know more about managing stress. To feel well, people must arrange their lives so as to satisfy certain basic needs. These needs may be physical, emotional, intellectual, creative, social, or existential. Knowing about these basic needs and satisfying them can lead to mental health that is relatively free of undue stress. Therefore, to approach life with the best possible chance of minimal stress, the needs that are most important to an individual must be met on a regular basis. At the end of this chapter, I will describe various techniques that anyone can use to cope with stress that occurs despite his or her best efforts to avoid or prevent it.

Physical Needs

It sometimes amazes me how little attention people pay to the obvious physical needs that we all have as human beings. We can observe this phenomenon in every crowd—in people who are grossly over-weight, undernourished, or looking much older than their years.

In this affluent country, there is either too much time spent on diet and food or not enough. I will not discuss in this chapter the need for adequate food intake free of excessive fats or sweets. Most of us know what we should be eating and what we should avoid. It is not a question of ignorance with most of us, but a lack of determination to treat our bodies in a way that would produce optimal health. We simply cannot drink 10 cups of coffee or a dozen Cokes a day and feel calm. Caffeine is a stimulant that produces uneasy feelings when taken in excess.

There is no doubt that emotional factors also play a large part in nutrition. Some people eat excessively when they are upset; others eat too little when under pressure.

It is quite clear that an adequate diet with vitamin and mineral supplements provides a good start toward feeling in control and free of stress. But it takes more than proper eating to feel well. Exercise is also important. Again, it is not out of ignorance that most of us do not exercise. We offer many rationalizations: "I have no time," "It's too hard," "I walk a lot at my work," or "I play golf once a week" (which usually means riding in a cart rather than walking). But everyone knows that regular exercise is good for the body and for the soul. Our bodies are made to move and to do so with some regularity. It is important to our emotional health to keep muscles and joints moving. Exercise also improves the circulation and generally fosters good health.

Because all of these benefits are so obvious, why do so few people exercise? Partly, the reason is cultural. We are now witnessing changes in attitude toward exercise, especially among the young. When it becomes the in thing to do and is more socially acceptable, it is easier for the average person to engage in a desirable activity. In Europe, people ride bicycles frequently. In our country, until recently, a person had to be a real individualist or a character to ride a bike in the neighborhood. As exercising becomes more fashionable, more people do it. We have to lay aside rationalizations about exercise and plan a regular time to do an aerobic activity, one that gets the heart beating at a higher rate than normal for 20–30 minutes several times per week. If we complain about feeling stressed, we should begin with a regular program of exercise. An exercise program does not solve all stress problems, but it is a good start. (Everyone should check with a physician first to make sure that an exercise regimen is suitable for his or her physical condition.)

Emotional Needs

Our emotional needs vary somewhat from one person to another. However, most of us have needs that are remarkably similar. We all need companionship of some kind. We all need to express our anger at times. We all need to laugh at ourselves periodically. Furthermore, we need work that is significant to us, work that has some meaning. Most of us need to be needed.

Aren't all these needs obvious? Yes, but so often I see individuals who are out of tune with their emotional needs. For example, Joe has a need for a companion, but somehow he always seems to find a person with whom he interacts badly, someone who does not meet Joe's emotional needs. He feels angry and overreacts, expressing the anger in a way that it is ineffective in dealing with his friend. Or there's Mary, who has a superior intellect but never had the persistence to get a good education. She now finds herself in a job as a clerk-secretary. Such work is simple for her but fails to meet her emotional needs. There is little satisfaction for her in performing her work, even though she is quite capable of doing so.

It is easy to see how these individuals will experience stress. If they were able to figure out how they are not meeting their emotional needs, the stress would be diminished. A time for self-analysis may be all that is necessary to discover what has gone wrong. Sometimes a friend or relative can see the obvious and offer good advice. Often, however, such problems are not easily corrected. Some individuals need a psychotherapist to help decipher the nature of the problem and to lead them to a constructive solution.

Some people have a greater than average need to be with others. They cannot stand to be alone. If such individuals find themselves in an isolated situation, they may become unhappy. They might have to cultivate the ability to be alone for short periods of time. Others have a strong need to be alone for many hours or even days. Hermits get along well enough by themselves without much contact with others. Although hermits may be an exception, there are many who prefer to be alone rather than with people.

Intellectual Needs

I have known college-educated individuals who have few if any needs to use their brains for more than their jobs or their check-books. It is hard for me to imagine anyone who has gone through college who has not developed the need to read books and discuss these materials with others. One of the pleasures that I remember with fondness was belonging to a book discussion group consisting of people with varied backgrounds and professions. The group discussed an array of ideas that proved stimulating and provocative. One of the gifts of an education is the continual interest it provides in seeking ideas and information.

There are fascinating persons who have had little education but have managed to read a tremendous amount and become self-educated. An outstanding example is Eric Hofer, author of *The True Believer* and *The Ordeal of Change*. He was a longshoreman most of his adult life, but he read prodigiously and was completely self-educated.

I have known friends and patients who have developed an outstanding vocabulary and who read widely because of their intellectual interests. Some people have a sense of these needs but never seem to get around to doing anything about them. If you realize that you have intellectual needs and are not presently doing anything to satisfy these needs, it is vital that you do so. Perhaps you are curious about how things work, or you may have an interest in how humankind came to be on this earth. History, art, or psychology may have interested you in a fleeting way at one time, and you did not pursue this interest. Now may be the time to do just that. Join a book group or take courses at local colleges. You will be surprised how much it enriches your life and even increases your self-esteem. Becoming engrossed in intellectual pursuits also has a way of draining off excess stress. In part, it will help suppress conflicts and distract you from the problems of everyday life, in much the same way that music or art is able to do.

Creative Needs

Does everyone have creative needs? My guess is that we all have such needs to one degree or another. There are individuals I know who could not exist without doing something creative. They are true artists in their everyday lives, if not as professionals. They live and breathe creativity. For them, life would be empty if they did not have some way of expressing their needs. Some of us fail to see the beauty around us, the delightful mannerisms of a child, the beauty of a sunset, or even the beauty of rain, with its temporary inconvenience. When it snows, I hear many complain that it stops them from doing what they wish. To me, it's a pleasant and often beautiful diversion, if not an opportunity to enjoy skiing. When is the last time we noticed folds of snow on the roof or the delicate patterns that the weather plays on the snow after several days? As with other activities in life, we have to practice observing things; otherwise, we miss so much that is worthwhile. These really are aesthetic needs. As humans, we are uniquely capable of appreciating the aesthetic. What does this have to do with our creative needs? Artists are good observers. They appreciate the colors, the designs, and the nuances of things. They are experts in certain aesthetic aspects of life. Most of us do not create works of art, but that should not prevent us from appreciating the works that others have created. Even the quality of a fine suit or the material in a favorite dress can help remind us of our aesthetic nature. Thomas Moore, in an excellent book called *Care of the Soul: A Guide for Cultivating Depth and Sacredness in Everyday Life*, speaks of the need to attend to these details in our lives as part of the many aspects of care of the soul.

On the other hand, many individuals discover some hidden talent that has lain dormant for years because they kept telling themselves that they had no creative abilities. Then, one day the creative tug appears when a friend suggests an art class or a course in a manual craft. A whole new world opens up, and these individuals see things in a different light. Those involved in creative activities rarely complain that the activity itself causes them stress; rather, they speak of the stress-relieving nature of the activity. Thus, paying attention to their creative needs does much to prevent or diminish the stress that may be present. I know physicians who are amateur artists. Some began their art careers while still working full-time as physicians. Other did not get involved in art until they retired. Yet, these creative activities produced many soul-pleasing experiences for these amateur artists and those around them.

Shortly after finishing my medical school training, as the pace of life slowed down for a time, I was surprised to find that I could enjoy drawing and painting, activities that I had never previously done. Although I do not possess great skill in the world of art, the work that I was able to complete did contribute to an entirely new period of relaxation for me. Although I have not pursued these activities vigorously, I can always return to drawing and painting if I wish to do so.

Social Needs

Some people have extraordinary needs to be around others. They cannot be alone for any length of time without, for example, talking on the telephone or going to the supermarket to see other people. Others do with much less socializing. Although there is wide variation in the amount of people contact needed between these two extremes of socializing, it is certain that the interaction that goes on among people and their friends is not just a simple need to socialize. It is a biological, emotional, and mental necessity. As an example, it has been shown that infants can become severely withdrawn or even die, not because they do not receive enough food but because they do not receive the caressing and holding that they require. This finding was reported based on observations made in South American orphanages where there was extremely limited care given to the infants.

The need for socialization in adults also is evident. Failure to interact sufficiently with others can bring on depression and other emotionally induced symptoms, which are especially evident among the older retired population. As evidence to support this idea, it has been shown in animal experiments that elderly rats continue to grow nerve tissue when exposed to socialization. Failure to socialize results in nerve deterioration, nerve cell death, and premature aging. The same phenomena are observed in the behavior of older adult humans. Experiments conducted at the Columbia University College of Physicians and Surgeons in New York show that when a nerve is stimulated, it actually sends out new branches (dendrites) to other nerve cells. There is a definite relationship between the degree of activity and socializing that is done by an older person and the maintenance of good levels of mental alertness, as well as physical and emotional health. Isolation and the lack of interaction with others on a regular basis contribute to deterioration of mental, physical, and emotional health.

We all have social needs, some more so than others. But if we have not paid attention to these needs, then it is time to begin. Without being with others, most of us would deteriorate over time. To reduce stress, it is important to be with those people who have interests that are similar to ours and who can discuss mutual interests with us.

Existential Needs

How do we view the world? What makes it tick for us? What is the purpose of it all? These are questions about our very existence. We all have different answers, and our views have much to do with how we handle stress. For example, someone who has a strong religious faith often can overcome illness and stress that may be much bigger problems to another person who does not have the backup of faith that God will see him or her through, come what may. The believer does not always request that God make the stress go away; rather, he or she asks to get through the difficult period in his or her life with the support and confidence that a strong faith allows. It is certainly difficult to know just how much a strong faith matters. It depends to a great degree on the mental state of the person. For example, when in a deep depression, it is difficult for depressed individuals to really believe that anything will ever get better. When in a panic attack, most people cannot use their faith effectively. But during less severe times, prayer or meditation is more effective than during the overwhelmingly stressful times. It is my observation that religious faith can be extremely effective in dealing with chronic disease states. Alcoholics Anonymous uses it effectively. Patients can achieve a degree of serenity and control over their illness and life through the use of their faith.

Probably all of us have heard these expressions: Don't sweat the small stuff, followed by Everything is small stuff! and Go with the flow. These are useful thoughts for anyone who is under stress to remember. They represent a way of looking at the world. Is it not remarkable how on any given day the events we are involved in are *the* most important to us? We need to look back at the things we were stressed by 10 years ago and try to visualize why we were so upset. Or we could even look at yesterday. Few things, in retrospect, seem as stressful as they were at the time we were going through them. We get all too involved in the "small stuff." We often lose the big picture and concentrate on the minutiae of life.

When I think about life, a metaphor comes to my mind. I think of a river. I see too many of my patients and friends swimming upstream instead of going with the flow of life. I see too many persons hung up on the rocks in the river. I see individuals caught up in the turbulence of the rapids instead of thinking of the calm wide waters that follow. Occasionally, I have remarked to patients who are going through one of life's reality crises, "This too shall pass." We have to see life in proper perspective—not an easy task. I certainly have not always done so successfully. It also is important to remind myself of my own advice from time to time. Life, as with a profession, demands that we *practice* it.

It has been curious to me that many people do not seem to need an existential view of life. They go on from day to day and are not troubled with the big picture. For them, if their daily needs are met, they see themselves progressing along life's path without too much difficulty. They appear to be content in avoiding asking what life is all about. Or, somewhere in the past, they have laid these questions to rest with the thought, I can't figure that out, and I'm not going to worry about it. But for others, it is important that some answers be found. If we are bothered by existential matters, we should continue our search but not when we are highly troubled, especially when we are in a deep depression. Answers generally are not found at such a time. We must wait until the crisis is over before pursing life's meaning.

Before wondering what to do about specific stresses that we experience, we should consider our basic needs. If we think about our needs and do our best to meet them, our stress will be far less than if these needs are not met. It is tragic, for example, to see persons involved in work that does not suit their needs or to see those who obviously need exercise but do not take a few minutes each day to meet their requirements for physical activity.

What to Do About Stress Now

Anyone can follow the next six suggestions to help alleviate stress:

1. Get the proper amount of sleep that you require. Most people need 6–8 hours of sleep per night. Don't make yourself an exception to this guideline unless it has been a lifelong pattern with which you are familiar. I know a few friends who sleep about 4 hours each night but are extremely productive during the day and are not known for their complaints about stress. They are the exceptions.

2. See to it that you obtain a significant amount of exercise at least three times per week. Jogging 10 miles a day is not necessary and often is physically harmful, especially to older individuals. Regular exercise is more important than intense workouts. Don't rationalize the need for exercise. Plan it as part of your schedule.

3. The importance of good nutrition cannot be overemphasized. Fad diets are of little value. The most important thing to do is avoid fatty foods and sweets. Good nutritional guidelines are available in books and from the American Heart Association.

4. Relaxation training techniques are available on audiotapes (e.g., from Effective Learning Systems, Inc., 5221 Edina Boulevard, Edina, Minnesota 55439). A large number of tapes are available on topics such as managing stress and deep relaxa-

tion. The tapes are of good quality and are inexpensive—about $10 each. Others may prefer meditation in one form or another. I do not believe that the method used is important. The regular practice of meditation can be beneficial in reducing stress.

5. Pay attention to your physical, emotional, intellectual, creative, social, and existential needs. They are all important. Individuals who function well usually have attended to these needs and have worked them out to a satisfactory level.

6. Aside from these specific suggestions, I feel it is most important for you to take some time out during the day to be alone—to contemplate, think, feel. The old adage about taking time to smell the roses is good advice. Most people say that they don't have the time to do so, but a careful analysis of the way people spend time suggests that many opportunities are lost because of the lack of determination to do what needs to be done to reduce stress. Destructive habits get in the way, but if there is a true desire to change, it is quite possible to do so. The current saying, Just do it, may seem simplistic, but there are times in life when it is necessary to just do it.

PART II

HOW
EMOTIONAL ILLNESS
DIFFERS FROM
MENTAL ILLNESS

CHAPTER 6

ADJUSTMENT DISORDERS

Most of us at one time or another have been so greatly upset that we have experienced the sensations felt by those who have emotional illnesses, generally referred to as the neuroses. The difference between what healthy persons feel and what those who have neuroses feel is in the severity and the duration of the symptoms. For example, a healthy person may feel a momentary abnormal fear, whereas the phobic patient, when exposed to a phobic situation, feels extremely frightened and is unable to function for some time. Also, persons who have neuroses may appear healthy and behave normally in most ways, except under certain circumstances to which they are sensitized.

When a neurosis is present, it causes mild to moderate psychic pain or discomfort—symptoms of one kind or another. As a result of these disturbances, there usually is some interference with interpersonal relationships. There may be a mild, temporary disturbance in the ability to deal with reality. For example, people with phobias do not deal with reality as well as others do. Also, according to psychodynamic theory, neurotic behavior is thought to be due to a mental conflict. It was Freud's formulation that the basic biological impulses that we all possess (id) are in opposition to the conscience (superego). The self (ego) is supposed to arbitrate between these forces. If the id and superego are thus kept in balance, the mind is free of conflict. Various defense mechanisms aid in this process. A common defense, called repression, forces conflicts into the unconscious where they are temporarily forgotten. However, when repression or other defense mechanisms fail, according to Freud, the conflicts cause anxiety. He went on to call this condition the anxiety neurosis, which he said was the primary neurosis. In addition to anxiety, certain types of depression, psychosomatic symptoms, phobias, and other distressing disorders may occur.

But how do emotional disorders differ from mental disorders, commonly called *psychoses?* First of all, the psychoses are much more severe. They cause major, abnormal changes in thinking, feeling, and behavior. Individuals who have acute psychoses can be identified by their strange mannerisms, inappropriate dress and behavior, abnormal thought processes, or abnormal ways of expressing feelings. Those who have these disorders often withdraw from others and have poor interpersonal relationships. They are out of contact with reality and express severe distortions in thought, such as delusions (false ideas not common to the culture), or experience hallucinations (hearing voices or seeing visions). Frequently, there are mood disturbances with severe depression, elation, or manic behavior. In the physically caused (organic) type of psychosis, disorientation, short- or long-term memory defects, and impaired judgment also occur.

Patients often speak of fears that their neurotic behavior will escalate into a psychosis. This rarely happens because there generally is not a continuum from emotional illness to psychosis; that is, someone suffering from an anxiety neurosis or panic attacks does not one day become psychotic. Rather, individuals who experience a psychotic breakdown may feel stressed, but they have few if any preliminary symptoms suggesting a neurotic disorder. The psychosis may appear abruptly or gradually but does not evolve from a neurosis.

Both neuroses and psychoses can be either acute or chronic; they can be transient or last for years. I have seen people go through a psychotic reaction in as little as 24 hours, without ever having the incident recur, even after many years of follow-up. Others may have chronic disorders, such as schizophrenia, which can last a lifetime. The same is true of the neuroses.

Adjustment Disorders

Adjustment disorders are the most common of the emotional illnesses. Most of us probably have experienced an adjustment disorder at one time or another, when we had symptoms of depression, anxiety, overactivity, or withdrawal from our usual activities. I am certain that I have had adjustment reactions more than once in my life, such as reactions to the stress of being in medical school or having major surgery to replace a defective heart valve. At these times, anxiety or psychosomatic symptoms occurred for short periods. As the stress was relieved, the symptoms vanished. These same stressors would not necessarily affect everyone in the same way. For example, many of my classmates in medical school did not seem particularly stressed.

I have seen patients undergo adjustment reactions because of impending marriage, divorce, loss of a job, or loss of a loved one or because of any of life's nerve-racking experiences.

To qualify as an adjustment disorder, the symptoms that occur must result from psychological stressors lasting at least 3 months, and they may not persist for more than 6 months. It is also essential that there is no other detectable psychiatric disorder. To qualify as an adjustment disorder, however, the reaction to the stressor has to be greater than usually is seen in the general population; the person has to have a certain degree of dysfunction, if only temporarily.

According to DSM-IV, the adjustment disorders are subdivided as follows:

- With depressed mood
- With anxiety
- With mixed anxiety and depressed mood
- With disturbance of conduct
- With mixed disturbance of emotions and conduct
- Unspecified

As can be seen from the types of adjustment disorders listed, the symptoms can manifest themselves in various ways, and although they appear self-explanatory, the following case example may help to clarify them.

Case Example

With the downturn in the economy in the United States during the late 1980s and early 1990s, many individuals lost their jobs either temporarily or, in many cases, permanently. When the loss of a job occurs in a young person's life, it can be difficult, but when it happens to older persons, who have a great deal of responsibility, it can have a profound effect.

My patient, John, lost his job at age 51. He had three children in college, and his wife worked part-time. He was optimistic, at least for the first month or two. He felt confident in his abilities and had little doubt that he would be working soon. But after 4–5 months, when no sign of a new job appeared on the horizon, panic set in. A period of depression followed, mixed with anger. It was obvious to John and his wife that he required treatment because he was not in any condition to go for job interviews. After a period of psychotherapy and medication, lasting for 2 months, John was able to function well again, and he went on to obtain employment.

Most people handle adjustment disorders without professional assistance. Friends, relatives, and confidants make suggestions, give support, and are available to see the individual through the crisis. They can be helpful just by listening and being a sounding board for the distressed person. An outsider can usually see things in a more optimistic manner, although it usually is not helpful to be overly optimistic with someone in distress. Excessive optimism tends to turn off the person who is going through a period of adjustment. The person with an adjustment problem certainly should try to relieve stress by the ways mentioned in Chapter 5 in this volume (e.g., meditation, relaxation techniques, and exercise). But for those who suffer from undue anxiety, depression, unusual conduct, or psychosomatic symptoms, it may be necessary to seek professional help. By definition, adjustment disorders are of short duration and therefore do not require any prolonged treatment. Short-term therapy can be valuable; often it will ward off more serious difficulties.

Psychosomatic Disorders

Physical complaints can be troublesome for some people. If physical symptoms are transient, they are of little concern to the average individual. But there are times when complaints about physical symptoms are prolonged and become psychosomatic illnesses. Strictly speaking, these illnesses are not adjustment disorders but may grow out of chronic stress. Nevertheless, I discuss several common psychosomatic disorders in this chapter. Other disorders, such as those of eating and sexuality, which also are regarded as psychosomatic, warrant discussion in separate chapters.

Psychosomatic disorders are the result of unresolved mental conflicts and their effects on our bodies. When a conflict occurs, some people handle it easily, whereas others regard the conflict as a major concern. At first, it may have a mild effect on the body—on a particular organ system. If the conflict is brief, no real damage occurs to the affected organ, such as the stomach or intestinal tract. But if the conflict is more chronic and persistent, a physical disease will result, such as stomach ulcers, colitis, or skin ailments.

Why do some people get psychosomatic illnesses and others seem to go through life without them? The exact answer to this question is not known. However, certain theories have been suggested. One old notion is that most of us have a "weak organ." That is, given enough stress, we feel it somewhere in our bodies. Some get stomachaches; others get headaches, skin rashes, or heart palpitations. One organ system or another is affected. To me, this is a common-sense idea. I believe it is true for me, as well as for the many patients with whom I have talked over the years. There is little doubt that we are born with certain physical and mental strengths and weaknesses that are determined by genetics. How we handle these various inborn qualities, in conjunction with our environment, determines what we become as persons. Some unfortunate individuals have many weaknesses, both physical and mental. Others are blessed with strong constitutions.

There was another older theory that certain personality types were strongly associated with the various psychosomatic illnesses.

Some physicians believed that there was an ulcer type of personality or an obesity or migraine type. However, in recent years this theory largely has been discounted, except for the link between heart attacks and the so-called type A personality. A series of studies done on heart attack patients showed that a surprising number of these patients have similar personalities. They are aggressive, driven individuals obsessed with time and impatient with those who do not move as quickly as they do. For example, they are known to finish sentences for others in conversations. The whole world does not move fast enough for them, whether in traffic, at work, or in relationships with others. Type A persons try to do three things at once (e.g., eating, reading, and watching TV). They find it hard to relax. They are self-serving and do not look out for others. Type A people like to acquire things, whether it is property, money, or any other show of success.

Efforts have been made to change these personality traits by means of individual and group therapy. Such treatments have met with success in motivated patients, although it is not easy to alter type A personalities. These individuals can learn to slow down, be less aggressive, and be more concerned about and compatible with others.

It seems that patients with psychosomatic disorders, with the exception of those with type A personality, generally do not express their emotions as well as most others do. They are too agreeable, ingratiating, and accepting of difficulties. Many psychotherapists believe that these traits are conducive to the evolution of psychosomatic illnesses. However, there are exceptions. We all know individuals who do not express their feelings well and yet do not necessarily have psychosomatic ailments.

Recently, emphasis has been placed not on personality traits or types but on the emotional situation that the person experienced just before the onset of his or her psychosomatic disorder. For example, if a man had severe job conflicts or was fired from his job and then developed a physical disorder, the emotional climate of his job and the nature of his conflicts at that time would be important issues on which to concentrate. Resolving these issues would help to solve the psychosomatic problems that ensued.

Stomach and Duodenal Ulcers

The medical world does not know the exact cause of ulcers. It has been presumed for some time that whatever causes ulcers to develop, emotional factors play a large part in the onset and even the prolongation of these diseases. However, even the treatment of ulcers has changed greatly since I went to medical school. Formerly, bland diets and mild food products were highly recommended, but now these are discouraged. New drugs have been extremely successful in treating ulcers in a short period of time. More recently, there was a report that the cause of stomach ulcers was a bacterium that responded to an antibiotic. I think it is obvious that the last word on these diseases has not yet been written. In the meantime, most physicians seem to agree that the emotional life of patients who have ulcers is important in aggravating the condition, if not in causing the problem.

No psychiatrist whom I know would presume to treat stomach or duodenal ulcers with psychotherapy alone. It is customary to work with a physician who is familiar with the current treatment of the disease. Dealing with the emotional factors and the physical ailment provides the optimal means toward cure.

Case Example

A 35-year-old man, Will, was referred to me by his internist. He had stomach ulcers that were clearly visible on X rays. The emotional problems, about which the internist was aware, mostly involved Will's job. Will complained of a strident boss who was on his back all the time. Will had asked his internist if he should quit his job and look for another. His physician wisely told him that he did not think that he could advise him on such an important matter. The internist suggested that he consult with me on the matter. When I inquired into the job conflict, it appeared that my patient had a definite problem in clearly expressing his feelings with his boss. It was true that Will's supervisor was overbearing, but others did not experience him this way all the time. They seemed to handle him better by asserting themselves. When I asked Will about his marriage, it was apparent that he had the same conflict there. His wife was slightly aggressive, and he felt put down by her. Unable to confront her with his feelings directly, he turned his anger inward, became somewhat depressed, and developed ulcers.

Fortunately, Will was amenable to change. Gradually, he learned to be more assertive both at work and at home. As a result, he began to feel much better about his job and his marriage. It took about 6 months for him to resolve his emotional problems. In the meantime, new X rays revealed that his stomach ulcer had healed and he no longer suffered from pain.

In this case example, the combination of medical and psychiatric treatment led to the best care of the patient. It was also important for the patient to be aware of his emotional conflicts and to know how to deal with them. With his newfound knowledge of how his emotional life affected his body, he was capable of preventing future physical problems.

Colitis

Colitis is an inflammation of the intestinal tract. The types, causes, and treatments of colitis are beyond the scope of this chapter. Regardless of the diagnosis, whether spastic colitis, ulcerative colitis, or any other form, it is generally agreed that emotional factors play a large part in either causing or aggravating this condition. There is little doubt that many other factors, such as heredity, diet, and infection, are involved in causing colitis; some factors have yet to be discovered.

Persons who have colitis often are limited in what they can do. I have met salespeople who can go only a certain distance from home before they experience severe abdominal cramps. They have to stop what they are doing and then find the nearest rest room for relief. There are businesspeople who cannot sit through a 2-hour meeting without recurrent abdominal distress. These same individuals are quite comfortable when they are relaxing at home.

The emotional conflicts surrounding those who have colitis are not easily uncovered. For some reason, psychosomatic disorders are firmly entrenched in the body, and rooting out the contributing emotional causes is not an easy matter. The most important factor involved is the defense of denial. This mental mechanism makes it possible for individuals with the illness to tell themselves that there are no conflicts and that their problems are purely physical. These individuals pursue medical cures without giving any thought to the possibility that emotional problems may be present in their lives. There are physical and medical dimensions to all psychosomatic illnesses, but these are relatively easy to handle. As a result, patients with colitis often do not seek the help of a psychiatrist in conjunction with the treating internist or family practitioner. However, when the psychiatrist is involved, the potential for better treatment results exists. Furthermore, if patients are aware of their emotional conflicts and learn to deal with them successfully, they can hope to ward off future attacks of this distressing disorder. Incidentally, colitis is sometimes associated with depression, usually of a mild to moderate type. I have found that in treating patients who have depression with coexisting colitis, their colitis improved. In part, this improvement may have been due to improvements in these patients' emotional lives, but it also is related to the fact that antidepressants have a quieting effect on the intestinal tract. Some patients experience complete cessation of their colitis when taking certain kinds of antidepressants.

Headaches

Among the many reasons for people getting headaches are tension, trauma, migraine, sinusitis, infections, high blood pressure, allergies, toxins, and any growth within the brain (tumors) or the tissues covering the brain. There are other reasons for the occurrence of headaches, but they are rare. Tension and migraine are by far the most common causes of headaches. The remaining causes are usually specific biological or organic problems, of which headache is one part of a cluster of symptoms. In psychosomatic disturbances, tension headaches stand out as the one ailment known to everybody. Migraine is less common, although we all know someone who has the condition.

Case Example

After a hard morning of work, my patient, Bob, notices that he has a headache in the usual places: over his forehead and in the back of his neck. He can feel the muscle tension in his neck on one side or the other, sometimes on both. Although he is aware that his work brings on the tension, he always seems at a loss to know what to do about it. When he discussed the problems he has at work, Bob became aware of his overreaction to some of his co-workers. Certain people regularly aroused his anger by their comments or ways of working. It was predictable. By 10 or 11 o'clock in the morning he could count on a headache. Although aspirin or other pain relievers helped, by midafternoon the headaches returned. In contrast, he seldom had headaches on weekends.

After a period of reflection on his problem, Bob learned how to modify his characteristic response to the people at work, and his headaches became less frequent. However, he also had to learn other means of dealing with the symptoms. I taught him how to relax his neck muscles with hot showers, neck rotation movements, and general relaxation exercises. By so doing, he was able to prevent the typical reactions to the job stress and interrupt the symptoms if they did recur.

With psychosomatic illnesses, the patient and the physician cannot hope to obtain absolute cure in the sense that the patient never has a recurrence of symptoms. In Bob's case, reducing the frequency of the headaches to a minimum, shortening the time of the headaches, and gaining some control over their occurrence were considered by Bob to be reasonable goals.

Migraine headaches are only partially psychosomatic. The first fact to note is that migraine tends to run in families. It is uncertain whether migraine is directly inherited, but there is usually a family history of migraine in a patient's mother, father, or other close relative. There are other differences in migraine that are specific for this form of headache. These headaches usually occur on one side of the head, with throbbing and pain mostly behind the eye. Nausea and vomiting are commonly associated with migraine.

I rarely have had patients come to me just for the treatment of migraine. Most of the patients with this disorder have come with other symptoms such as depression or anxiety.

Case Example

Jane had the typical family history, with both her mother and aunt suffering from migraine. Jane's attacks occurred about 1–2 months apart. Sometimes they were preceded by an unusu-

ally busy but productive day. Often, the headaches followed a period of tension. When they happened, Jane was "down for the
count" for about 2 days with her "sick" headache. Usually, it subsided after she had an episode of vomiting. Jane knew that some of
her emotional problems contributed to the migraine. But it was
even more obvious that her depression was the direct result of her
conflicts.

Curious things happen in the practice of medicine. Often, in
treating one illness, a second one also gets better, as with colitis and
depression. Such was the case with Jane. When her depression was
treated with medication and psychotherapy, her migraines all but
disappeared. Just why her migraine headaches improved is not exactly known, but it has been observed that certain antidepressant
medications seem to block migraine attacks. When the antidepressants are discontinued, the migraine is apt to return.

From a practical point of view, I do not think it is worthwhile to
engage patients in long-term psychotherapy for the specific treatment of migraine. Nor have I ever heard of good research studies that
indicated that migraine should be treated by psychotherapy alone. It
is my opinion, that as with all psychosomatic disturbances, the best
results are obtained by a combination of medication and psychotherapy. Probably most migraine patients are treated by family physicians
or internists with the old medical remedies, which abort the migraine, and some newer medications, which are reported to prevent
the attacks. An injectable form of medication is also available for the
treatment of migraine.

Skin Diseases

Although many skin diseases have psychosomatic aspects, I focus on
only three of them in this discussion: urticaria (hives), neurodermatitis, and atopic dermatitis (eczema).

Under stress, some individuals get blotchy skin, with round or irregular red areas that are commonly called hives. These rashes are inflamed and raised, and they tend to itch severely. The stress can be of
any kind, but it often is due to interpersonal stress. Patients who have
this form of dermatitis usually are quite aware of the situations that

bring on the hives. As with most diseases, there are many causes for the symptoms. Allergies are probably the most common reason for hives, but when allergies are eliminated as the prime problem, a psychosomatic cause is assumed. Various local remedies such as hydrocortisone ointments or creams are helpful in treating these disorders, but attention to the conflicts that patients experience when they have hives also is important in preventing and eliminating the disease.

Neurodermatitis consists of localized areas of dry, scaly, itchy skin. One or more patches may exist and appear to break out during periods of stress. Related to this condition, but of a more generalized nature, is the disease atopic dermatitis, or eczema. The dry, itchy rash is usually found on the arms, legs, and face, but when the symptoms flare up badly, especially in the winter season, it can involve almost the entire skin surface. As a child and young adult, I was all too familiar with this condition. I was told that the eczema affected me even as an infant, and I was aware of the discomfort and itching throughout my childhood. In college, it was particularly bad. It was clear to me that warm weather and the lack of stress had a good effect on the condition. At one point, I was advised to go to a warm climate. A year at college in Arizona resulted in a remarkable improvement in the eczema. Later, while going through medical school, the symptoms were at their worst. These were the days before cortisone preparations were readily available. Dermatologists had other remedies at the time, but they were not helpful.

Eczema is a disease that has allergic elements. It tends to run in families. It often clears up in adult life. Fortunately, as I aged, the dermatitis virtually disappeared. I credit this in part to the aging process, although aging does not help everyone who has the disease. I also think that my training as a psychoanalyst, and especially the requirement that I undergo a period of personal psychoanalysis, was responsible for eliminating many of the emotional aspects of this condition. It is a genuine pleasure to have normal, healthy skin after many years of discomfort and embarrassment.

To treat dermatitis, remedies prescribed by a dermatologist are usually sufficient, but when obvious emotional factors are involved, psychotherapy is helpful in resolving the emotional component of the illness.

As with adjustment disorders, persons who have psychosomatic disorders do not always go to psychiatrists for treatment, nor is it always necessary. It depends on the severity of the symptoms and the duration of the problem. If the treating physician can handle the situation and successfully eliminate the symptoms, psychotherapy is not necessary. However, if the illness is overwhelming and chronic, psychotherapy should be considered.

What Can Families, Friends, and Caregivers Do?

Caregivers should be aware that adjustment disorders are of short duration and are usually brought on by external events. As such, these disorders require support and understanding from family, friends, and caregivers for only a short time. But if such help is not forthcoming, the condition can be prolonged. Specific advice by caregivers often is not appreciated. Some understanding and comfort help more.

Persons with psychosomatic disorders are particularly prone to deny any psychological causes for their illnesses. Caregivers can firmly suggest that psychological factors may be present and give examples of how this may be true. It is difficult to get these individuals to consider treatment from psychotherapists, but family and friends should try to do so, particularly if the individuals have obvious conflicts in their lives that need attention.

CHAPTER 7

THE NEUROSES

There are many ways in which a neurosis can manifest itself in our lives. It may appear as a phobia, a physical symptom, or extreme apprehension, or it may appear in more unusual ways. Some of my patients have had multiple symptoms.

Case Example

Janet was 35 years old and single. She came to see me because of overwhelming anxiety, which was beginning to interfere with her life. Janet appeared to be a healthy vivacious person, but she was overcome by her symptoms. For about 3 months, she had noticed that when she awakened in the morning, she did not feel well. She felt a tension in her body, abdominal cramps, and a vague feeling of apprehension. As she prepared to go to work, she felt even worse. When at her job, tasks that ordinarily would be routine for her seemed to bring on much more tension. She also noticed that on the way home from work, she felt much better, although the tension and anxiety lingered. Janet had trouble going to sleep, but once asleep, she did well until the next morning. Occasionally, she had dreams that were disturbing.

When Janet tried to alleviate her anxiety, nothing seemed to help her much except a hot bath or some exercise. I asked myself the question, Why did Janet develop these particular symptoms at this particular time? In the preceding years, she had enjoyed good emotional and physical health. What was going wrong now? I explored the past with Janet. She came from a home of successful people. Her father was a businessman who had worked his way from poverty to the head of a small but thriving enterprise. Her mother was a nurse, quite able to work long hours in a busy hospital. Her siblings were also doing well. Her older sister was a college graduate, now married and working part-time. Her younger brother became an attorney, was married, and appeared to be happy with his life.

Furthermore, I learned that Janet had worked hard in school and had obtained a graduate degree in business. She was now earning a good income and was financially secure. Although she liked her job, her boss was harassing her more and more, and she did not feel effective in stopping him. She lived alone in an apartment, had a number of good friends, but had been notably unsuccessful in her love relationships. Two long-term affairs had ended in rejection by her lovers. More recently, her current male friend was showing signs of disinterest. Janet had dreamed that once she had been successful in establishing her career, she would likely marry and perhaps have children. She was beginning to have some doubts about these possibilities. She had read in women's magazines many articles about careers and marriage and how to combine the two commitments. Now she was having trouble reaching some of her long-range goals.

The initial symptoms of anxiety and insomnia that Janet spoke about responded well to some mild antianxiety medication. However, her encroaching conflicts were not so easily resolved. We had to spend some weeks trying to get a grasp on what was bothering her. She was a hardworking, trusting person who had given much of herself to her job and her personal relationships. The people in her life had not always responded in kind. For example, she found herself frequently doing more for her close friends than they did for her. She was more thoughtful and caring and helpful to her friends than they were to her. At times, Janet felt the unfairness of these situations, but she rationalized the problem and gave other persons the benefit of the doubt. Occasionally, she felt some mild resentment toward her friends. Her boss asked her to do more than other employees at her level. He also was more than a little flirtatious with her. On two occasions, he asked Janet to go away with him on weekends, and when she refused, he badgered her about it. She felt that he was taking advantage of her good nature and stepping over the line on a personal level.

Janet had tried to be a "good girl" all her life. She succeeded in pleasing others well beyond what was required of her. Then, when people asked too much of her or disappointed her, she was unable to respond emotionally to them in ways appropriate to the situation. It took careful examination of her life for her to see that she was feeling quite hostile toward her male friend, her boss, and to a lesser degree her friends. Janet had denied her hostility, while she excused the behavior of those around her. Gradually, Janet was able to see clearly how she was trying too hard to please and was not being fair to herself in her relationships with others. It took some courage on her part to react differently. She had to learn to defend herself, stand up for her rights, and make clear her wishes. She had to risk the possible loss of some friendships. Actually, in time, her friends saw a new Janet that they liked even better. When Janet confronted her boss with her feelings, he backed off and was seldom a problem. When he did try to harass her again, she immediately reminded him of her feelings. This reminder put a damper on his aggressiveness; work no longer was a source of conflict.

Janet was able to see how her desire to please was a good trait that had been carried to excess. By modifying this behavior and asserting herself more, she was able to manage her life in a more satisfactory manner. Her male friend did not reject her, and within a short time, he began to speak seriously about their future, something that had not been mentioned before. Janet had gained control over her life. She no longer felt hostility toward those around her. Consequently, her anxiety diminished and was virtually absent.

What Causes Neuroses?

Although there is not universal agreement on how neurotic illnesses develop, there is general consensus that anxiety is at the root of all neuroses, and it is the result of mental conflict. This idea was first formulated by Freud.

How did Freud's theories come about? Toward the latter part of the 19th century, Freud, a Viennese neurologist, became interested in a phenomenon called *hysterical conversion*. In this condition, the patient had symptoms such as paralysis of limbs and the inability to speak, hear, or see, presumably because of emotional distress. A leading Parisian physician, Charcot, was treating patients for this disorder at his clinic. He used classical hypnosis and was able to "cure" his patients. However, the symptoms often returned. This fact intrigued Freud. He postulated that there was a conflict going on in the patient causing the symptoms.

In an attempt to reach the source of patients' conflicts, Freud encouraged his patients to lie on a couch and let their minds wander. Patients were told to "free associate"—say anything that came to mind. With free association, in addition to a patient's recollection of dreams, Freud obtained much information about the patient that the patient was not able to discuss in ordinary conversation. With the material that he gathered by this method, he postulated that there were conflicts brewing in the patient's mind that caused the hysterical symptoms. He visualized the person's conscious self (ego) constantly engaged in arbitration between the conscience (superego) of the patient and his or her basic instincts of sex and aggression (id). He said that as long as the patient's ego successfully was able to manage these conflicts, no symptoms of neurosis developed. Managing conflicts was accomplished by the mind unconsciously forgetting about the conflicts through the mental defense mechanism of repression. But if repression was only partial and the patient was not able to push the conflict into his or her unconscious, then symptoms resulted. Freud stated that anxiety neurosis developed in this manner; he called it the *primary neurosis*. He further stated that other neuroses employed more involved defense mechanisms and resulted in different symptoms. These defense mechanisms are noted in the following discussions on the various neuroses.

What types of neuroses are there? How do they manifest themselves? These disorders are now described under three different categories. The current classification in DSM-IV is divided as follows:

- The anxiety disorders (anxiety, phobic neuroses)
- The somatoform disorders
- The dissociative disorders (hysterical neuroses, dissociative type)

Anxiety Disorders

Anxiety is a feeling of apprehension, usually accompanied by uncomfortable physical symptoms. These symptoms include heart palpitations, shortness of breath, restlessness, and internal tension. Anxiety can come on suddenly or gradually and may be mild or severe. As previously mentioned, most psychotherapists believe that anxiety is the result of mental conflict. According to Karen Horney, one of the original post-Freudian psychoanalysts, concerns about *security* and the *satisfaction of basic needs* are especially important. When these needs are not met or are threatened, the individual develops symptoms of anxiety.

In the case example at the beginning of this chapter, Janet felt extremely insecure when she could not please people. Her basic need to be loved and appreciated was in conflict with her feelings that people were taking advantage of her. Yet, she did not want to chance losing the security of those around her. When she was able to resolve these conflicts, her anxiety diminished.

We all suffer from some anxiety at one time or another. If the anxiety experienced is mild and transient, it is not called a neurosis; however, if the symptoms of anxiety are severe and persistent, then the resulting syndrome is referred to as a neurosis. There are various forms of neuroses.

Panic Disorder

Panic disorder is not a mild feeling of fright. It is a severe disturbance that is hard to endure. Patients who have this disorder sometimes feel like they are about to die. I can recall a young woman who told me about the first time she had a panic attack. Beth was sitting in a sports arena, high up in the balcony. About halfway through the basketball game, she became upset. Her heart began to pound, she could not catch her breath, and her fingers and toes had the sensation of pins and needles. The feeling was so overwhelming that she felt that she would not be able to make it out of the building, much less make it home. She begged her friend to take her out, but she felt faint, as though she would pass out. She had to sit down for a while before being able to proceed. On the way home she began to feel much relieved. Shortly after this event, she came to see me for treatment.

Often, after the first panic attack, patients like Beth fear a recurrence of the symptoms. The person feels increasingly uncomfortable when away from home, in public places, or in areas that are hard to leave, such as in traffic jams. When this fear of being in places or situations that are difficult to leave becomes a pattern, it is called *agoraphobia*. Some patients have only panic attacks. Others have panic attacks along with agoraphobia. Beth became agoraphobic after having several panic attacks.

One of the underlying problems present in patients with panic disorder with agoraphobia is the so-called separation anxiety. It may start in early childhood, when there is a fear of leaving the security of mother and home. It may occur in other forms later on. One example of this is school phobia, a common childhood fear. The fear can be about what might happen in school, but more commonly it is a fear of leaving the security of home.

In agoraphobia, the distance away from the source of security is of immense importance to patients suffering from this disorder. The further away from home they are, the more anxiety or panic occurs; the closer to home, the more relaxed they become. However, in some cases, panic attacks may occur even at home, when no obvious threat is present.

At times, agoraphobia can be so extreme that a person may fear leaving home because a panic attack may occur. I have seen such fear keep individuals home for months and even years. One of my patients had not left his home for several years until a physical emergency forced him to go to the hospital. This emergency broke the chain of fear, and from then on he was able to come to my office for treatment. Although it took considerable time, the patient did overcome both his agoraphobia and panic attacks.

In their need to maintain security, individuals who have agoraphobia commonly use the defense of avoidance. They avoid the places that are likely to bring on their symptoms. Panic attacks are extremely hard to endure. Most patients want immediate relief from the attacks. Attacks can be alleviated with appropriate medication. Currently, Xanax (alprazolam) or other antianxiety medications are used both to treat the panic and to prevent further attacks. But oddly enough, certain antidepressants are known to prevent panic attacks too. Medications such as Tofranil (imipramine), Elavil (amitriptyline), and Nardil (phenelzine) seem uniquely able to prevent panic attacks from occurring. With the protection of medication and the security that the panic attacks will not occur or will be mild, the patient is better able to look into the psychological aspects of these disorders. I generally recommend to patients that medication and psychotherapy be used at the same time. Beth, for example, did well with medication and psychotherapy. However, treatment was not quick because she had issues of separation anxiety that had to be addressed in order for her to feel entirely well.

There is now some evidence, based on imaging studies of the brain, that suggests a physical basis for panic disorders. Although this finding needs further confirmation, it is an interesting area of research. There is no doubt that biological and psychological factors play a part in the origin of panic and agoraphobia.

The families and friends of patients with panic disorder need considerable patience to deal with the insecurity of those who have panic attacks and agoraphobia. However, as with patients who have other phobias, patients with panic disorder or agoraphobia tend to use the defense of avoidance to a high degree. Those who are supportive of these patients should encourage them to fight their fears; medication also will help these patients to reach beyond what is feared. Too much empathy and understanding of the patients' fears on the part of caregivers can actually hinder progress.

Specific Phobia

There are many phobias that are familiar to everyone. Common types of phobias are fear of closed spaces (claustrophobia), heights (acrophobia), water (aquaphobia), fire (pyrophobia), strangers (xenophobia), dirt (mysophobia), and germs (microphobia). The object feared may be something that can be related to an earlier experience. For example, a phobia of boats may be connected to a near-drowning episode when someone was younger. Most of the time, however, a phobia has more symbolic significance, although frequently it is difficult to ascertain what the phobia represents.

Most psychiatrists will try to treat common phobias by gradually desensitizing patients to the feared object. For example, a person who is phobic of elevators may go with a therapist up one floor on an elevator and after repeated experiences may feel slightly more comfortable. After the patient successfully manages going up one floor, a trial of two floors is attempted. Gradually, the patient may become desensitized to the experience, and eventually he or she may go on an elevator alone. I have successfully treated patients with driving phobias by gradually having them drive farther with increasingly more traffic. After a time, they were satisfied that they could drive as far as they desired.

As with agoraphobia, the most common defense used by persons with common phobias is avoidance. By constantly avoiding the phobic object, these individuals actually increase their fear. But by gradually exposing themselves to the phobia in small increments, they often can learn to overcome it.

Social Phobia

As the term *social phobia* implies, people with this phobia are afraid to be in contact with groups. They become acutely embarrassed, are sensitive to criticism, and fear making errors in the presence of others. For these reasons, their lives are geared to avoiding any social situations. Some individuals with social phobia are able to go to a job and have limited contact with people. But it is difficult for them, and they retreat home as soon as possible. Emotionally, these people remain fearful and experience little joy. Here, too, gradual desensitization can prove helpful. Long-term psychotherapy is also of value.

Obsessive-Compulsive Disorder

Recurring intrusive thoughts (obsessions) and repeated actions (compulsions) that cannot be easily stopped characterize this condition. The thoughts may exist by themselves or may be followed or accompanied by compulsions. Compulsions involve ritualistic acts, which the person feels he or she must do to avoid anxiety. For example, a person may check the locks on his or her door 10 times at night before being completely certain that the door is locked. Even though the individual knows that the door is locked, he or she must check it again repeatedly; otherwise, he or she cannot go to sleep.

Every psychiatrist has seen patients with compulsive hand washing in which the person must wash his or her hands for a certain number of times. Only after that number has been reached can the individual stop and feel free of anxiety. If repetitive hand washing is not possible, the person experiences considerable anxiety. These symptoms are difficult to treat using only psychotherapy. I like to start treatment with some attempt at gradually decreasing the exact number of times the hands are washed. If the patient can stand the anxiety that follows, I ask him or her to decrease the hand washing further. If this technique does not work, I may prescribe one of the new medications that are known to interrupt obsessive-compulsive symptoms, such as Prozac (fluoxetine) or Anafranil (clomipramine).

I have seen a number of young mothers who had an obsession that they would harm their children in some way. For example, when passing through a doorway, the mother would be obsessed with the idea of hitting the baby's head on the doorpost. Although I have never seen or heard of such mothers ever harming a child, the very idea of it is frightening to these individuals. I have found that treatment for this form of obsession is usually brief, and that these patients respond well to psychotherapy, as illustrated in the following case example.

Case Example

Ruth was a young mother with a 2-month-old infant. She was trying hard to be a "good" mother. She had read several books on how to care for her child. So far, things had gone well. She felt that she was living up to her expectations as a mother and wife. At times,

she became overly tired because she worked too hard at being a du-
tiful person. Ruth did not allow much time to see her friends; her
baby was her main preoccupation. One day, she noticed that she
was becoming unusually afraid that something bad might happen
to her child, an event that she could not control. This worry was
tolerable. Ruth told herself that she was just a worrier and dismissed such thoughts from her mind as soon as she could.

Then, one day while cutting bread, she got the thought that she
would actually harm her child with the knife. The thought was so
overwhelming that Ruth immediately called her husband and
asked him to come home. While waiting for him, she decided to
throw the knife outside in the hope that she would not think about
it if it were out of sight. Meanwhile, she held on to her child, caressed him, and told him that she loved him. When her husband
came home, he found her in a distressed state. He had never seen
her like this before; he knew he had to get her help. After discussing the situation with the child's pediatrician, Ruth and her husband were referred to my office.

On the first visit to see me, Ruth appeared anxious. She talked
excessively and suddenly asked, "Am I going crazy? Will I have to
go to a mental hospital?" After carefully examining her, I was certain that she was suffering from an obsessive disorder. I reassured
her that she did not require hospitalization and that she was not
losing her mind. I also told her that the dreadful fear of harming
her child would not become a reality. I based this on my knowledge
and experience with such cases. Although she did not completely
believe me, Ruth became much calmer and relaxed. I told her husband about the nature of the problem and asked him to further reassure her about the obsession when he was at home.

As her psychotherapy progressed, it became apparent that
Ruth was working too hard at being a good mother. When her husband criticized her ever so slightly, she became upset and depressed about it. She had great difficulty expressing any anger
toward her husband, even about obvious sources of frustration for
her. I tried to help Ruth see the relationship between her obsession, her need to be "supermom," and her inability to express her
anger in appropriate ways. In effect, her repressed anger and frustration manifested themselves in a substitute form. Instead of being expressed appropriately toward her husband, her anger and
frustration were directed toward her child in the form of an obses-

sion. It took several months for this message to sink in, but Ruth gradually got in touch with her angry feelings and learned to express them in effective ways. With my assurance that Ruth would not harm her child and her newfound emotional insight, she was able to rid herself of the obsession and go on to be a mother in good control of her feelings. Meanwhile, her relationship with her husband improved as well.

Relatives, friends, and caregivers of persons with obsessive-compulsive disorder are often unsettled about how to deal with the problems of these individuals. Do I go along with all the compulsions? Do I listen to the constant obsessions? How can I remain empathic to the continual rumination and worry? The answers are not easy. First of all, it is important to be aware that the obsessions and compulsions are not fully under the control of the affected individuals. Much of their behavior is so emotionally driven that it is difficult to stop. However, it does not help if the family makes all kinds of concessions to the compulsive person. For example, giving in to a limited degree to someone's obsessive cleanliness makes sense, but the family should not become a slave to the obsessive-compulsive person in the household. Actually, when those surrounding the compulsive person continue to give in to the unreasonable demands to be compulsively clean, it can reinforce the person's need to be that way. On the other hand, if a relative insists that the compulsive person's behavior is "just crazy," it can only result in increased anxiety and tension between the two persons involved. A certain degree of understanding is helpful, but complete compliance to the illness is not. Rather, the family or friends should encourage the person to deal with the obsessive-compulsive behavior in a positive way.

Posttraumatic Stress Disorder

Posttraumatic stress disorder (PTSD) is a condition that follows severe disasters, such as earthquakes, hurricanes, or bombings, or the violence of murder, war, or accidents. By definition, the trauma must be severe. After the traumatic event, the person may experience anxiety, difficulty in concentrating, disturbing dreams, and a mental recurrence of the original trauma. Immediately after the traumatic episode, there usually is a *psychic numbing* in which there is a dissociation from the environment and an inability to deal with the normal requirements of the day. The person may appear to be in a daze and out of contact with reality. This numbing may last only a few hours or days, after which the individual may appear relatively normal, only to reexperience the trauma days or months later. There may be a partial or complete amnesia for the trauma, which can last for days or weeks. Events similar to the original trauma or anything that reminds the person of the catastrophic time may bring on the disorder. For example, Bill, a Vietnam veteran, witnessed the killing of his friends by bombs during the war and had a sudden dissociation from the experience. He was brought to a hospital for rest and soon recovered. But weeks later, Bill experienced severe reactions to any loud noise. On these occasions, he became overly anxious, perspired profusely, and had nightmares of the war.

PTSD was first recognized during World War II. It usually was observed in battlefield conditions. Soldiers were said to be suffering from shell shock. Anyone who has ever watched reruns of the TV series *M*A*S*H* probably has seen several episodes in which one of the characters is in a dazed state after being in the battlefield. The psychiatrist is called in to hypnotize him and give him an injection to help him come back to reality. These scenes depict what psychic numbing is and how psychiatrists handle the problem.

As another example, many victims of the Florida hurricane or the World Trade Center bombing will undoubtedly have PTSD. In recent years, PTSD has been too frequently used as a diagnosis for the anxiety that follows minor traumas such as car accidents. Although there may be some fear and anxiety about driving after an accident, these symptoms clearly do not fit the diagnosis.

Treatment of PTSD is best done by using psychotherapy and antianxiety medication. Sometimes hypnosis, with or without the use of a drug such as Amytal Sodium, is useful in helping the individual recall the forgotten events of the trauma, events that have been repressed into the unconscious. In addition to drugs, group therapy has been used effectively in treating this disorder.

Acute Stress Disorder

Patients with acute stress disorder have symptoms similar to those of PTSD that occur soon after a severe traumatic event.

Generalized Anxiety Disorder

In generalized anxiety disorder, excessive anxiety must be present for a period of at least 6 months and can vary in intensity. It is typical for those who have this condition to feel much more anxious about things than others do. Nervousness, excessive worry, apprehension, and increased physical stress are common. The internist or family physician should be aware that this disorder must be differentiated from diseases such as hyperthyroidism, hypoglycemia (low blood sugar), and certain neurological conditions.

Generalized anxiety disorder occurs in at least 5% of the population and is more common in females than males by 2 to 1. Treatment of this condition can be handled by psychotherapy and medication. It is one of the illnesses that is most responsive to psychotherapy and reassurance, although individuals with this disorder can become dependent on psychotherapists for relief of symptoms. There also is the risk of drug dependence in this group of patients. Some psychiatrists use behavioral or cognitive therapy to help ameliorate anxiety.

Other categories of anxiety disorders are the following:

- Anxiety disorder due to a general medical condition
- Substance-induced anxiety disorder
- Anxiety disorder not otherwise specified

Somatoform Disorders

Body Dysmorphic Disorder

Individuals with body dysmorphic disorder have a major preoccupation with a physical defect, which may be considered normal or hardly noticeable to the average viewer. Minor physical imperfections are given great importance by these patients. I have seen women who felt that their faces were permanently scarred by electrolysis. They saw huge pitting in the facial pores and other abnormalities where hair was removed. I had trouble seeing any of these defects even at close range. But it became a tremendous source of anxiety and a stated reason for lack of success in life. Similarly, patients with anorexia typically see themselves as fat, although any observer would view them as markedly underweight. This distortion in body image actually can be dangerous to the affected persons.

All of us are subject to some distortions of body image. We see ourselves in pictures somewhat different from what we see in the mirror. As one of my friends once remarked, "When I look in the mirror, I appear to have a full head of hair, but when I see pictures of myself, I realize how bald I am becoming."

Individuals who have body dysmorphic disorder are not easy to treat. Sometimes the distortions of body image are so severe that some patients feel hopeless; they may become depressed to the point of suicide. Psychotherapy is required for this condition, and it may be necessary to hospitalize some patients to stabilize them with medication and deal with their distorted thought processes. Body dysmorphic disorder can be a malignant condition, regardless of the form it takes. Reassurance by friends and family that the distortion of body image does not exist usually makes patients angry and seldom helps the situation. Professional help is important to prevent a serious outcome.

Conversion Disorder
(Hysterical Neurosis, Conversion Type)

It is interesting how illnesses change with the passage of time. When Freud started his work, conversion disorders were common. In Paris, there was an entire clinic set aside to deal with them. Today, they are rare. In more than 30 years of practice, I have seen perhaps a half dozen examples of this disorder. The following two case examples illustrate conversion disorder.

Case Example 1

I examined a young marine during my service in the United States Navy. He had done poorly in basic training, and he was placed in a retraining program. One day, he was required to go through an obstacle course. He resented this test, but his anger about it was mostly repressed, and he appeared to be compliant. He managed one obstacle after another and was about to climb a long rope when his hand became a clenched fist. He could not open it no matter how hard he tried. His sergeant yelled at him, but despite the anger of his superior, the marine was unable to open his fist. In disgust, the sergeant sent him to the physician at sick call with a few unkindly epithets. There the physician recognized the situation as a physical manifestation of a psychological problem and referred the marine to me for consultation.

When I saw him, the marine appeared nonchalant and unconcerned about his clenched fist. I gave him Amytal Sodium (for medical hypnosis) intravenously and told him that he could now open his fist and move his fingers spontaneously. He did so almost immediately. He and the other marines who were watching were amazed by the sudden "cure." However, it is typical in such cases that the symptoms soon return unless something is done about the underlying conflict that caused the physical abnormality. In this case, I was unable to follow through with the patient's treatment. If I had had the opportunity to do so, I would have pursued the meaning of the clenched fist—an obvious symbol of his repressed anger.

Case Example 2

I remember seeing a young woman who was paralyzed and unable to walk. She had collapsed suddenly after an episode with her boss during which he had yelled at her. Gail was brought to the emergency room of the local hospital where she was admitted to the orthopedic service. She had no orthopedic problem, so a neurologist was called in to examine her. He found no physical reason for her sudden paralysis and suggested a psychiatric consultation. When I saw Gail, she seemed to have little concern about her symptoms, a typical *la belle indifference* usually seen with this disorder. A colleague of mine was present in the hospital at the time. She was much more familiar with the technique of hypnosis than I, and I asked her to see the patient. While Gail was under hypnosis, the following story emerged: About a year ago, Gail's father had died, almost immediately after Gail and her father had argued. She felt guilty about this, and it had upset her for months. The anniversary of his death was approaching and her guilt was resurfacing. Then her boss confronted her about a minor mistake. She felt anger welling up in her but was unable to express her feelings. It was at this point that she collapsed and was unable to walk.

Gail's story is one of conflict in the classical tradition of Freud. It fit right into his theory of how neuroses develop. Gail's aggression, originating from the id, was in conflict with her superego. The patient was unable to repress the conflict sufficiently, and it came back with the anticipated anniversary of her father's death and the anger she felt with her boss. Her dramatic "paralysis" allowed her to escape the conflict and turn to the preoccupation with her physical concerns. During the hypnotic session, my colleague made the suggestion to Gail that there was nothing wrong with her physically, and that she could walk. She immediately stood up, walked around, and later was seen jumping up and down in the halls of the hospital. Gail was instructed to return for subsequent psychotherapy visits. After one visit, she failed to return and was not seen again. It is quite likely that her unresolved conflict would again produce another hysterical episode unless she sought help in dealing with her underlying conflict.

Somatization Disorder

In somatization disorder, there are many physical symptoms that preoccupy patients. The complaints may simulate cardiac, intestinal, orthopedic, neurological, or other problems. The symptoms exist without any true physical disease being detected. To qualify for this disorder, the symptoms must be numerous and be present for at least 2 years. The family practitioner and the internist treat many of these patients, and sometimes they refer them to psychiatrists when treatment proves unsuccessful, but these are difficult patients to help. They are so fixated on their physical symptoms that it is hard for them to think of anything else. Sometimes, given enough opportunity, the psychiatrist can get beyond the symptoms to underlying problems that these patients are not facing. We say that the anxiety is being somatized—put into physical form instead of being dealt with in a psychological sense. But by the time patients reach the psychiatrist, the pattern has become so set that recovery is difficult. However, if patients are truly motivated, much can be done to alleviate the preoccupation with bodily functions.

Hypochondriasis

Most people think that hypochondriasis is a preoccupation with illness, which is partially true. More specifically, hypochondriasis is a fear of having a serious disease, such as cancer, heart disease, or another major illness, that has lasted at least 6 months. The person seeks out one physician after another to try to confirm his or her suspicions that the disease actually exists. Despite elaborate diagnostic tests, no disease is found. Still not convinced, the person continues to visit physicians to confirm his or her "disease." Some patients insist on exploratory surgery to find the disease. When nothing is found, the person often believes that the physician was not skillful enough to find it.

Hypochondriasis is one of the more difficult psychiatric maladies to treat. Medications are of little help. There is such a major preoccupation with illness that the person has a hard time looking into the rest of his or her life for possible sources of conflict that may be responsible for the concerns. I once treated a middle-aged woman who felt she had heart disease. Every test available confirmed only that she was in good health. Despite her fear of heart trouble, she refused to take commonsense measures to avoid a genuine heart attack. She continued to smoke, did little or no exercise, and was careless about her diet. There also were a number of issues involving her husband and children, which clearly caused some of her emotional problems. In the process of psychotherapy, she learned to deal with these matters more appropriately, and gradually her concern with heart trouble diminished. Usually, the resistance to change is quite prominent with these patients. Many continue to believe that serious illness is present. Their belief often is so strong that it prevents them from looking into emotional reasons for the symptoms.

Pain Disorder

The perception of pain is unique to each individual. Some people are aware that they have a high pain threshold; that is, they are able to endure much more pain than the average person. Others can take little pain. Every dentist is familiar with this phenomenon.

Various situations have a powerful influence on pain. We all have had the experience of being in an accident that brings out the adrenaline and physiologically produced endorphins—the body's own painkillers. In such instances, we may endure a laceration or severe bruise and not feel it until the crisis is over. But when we anticipate pain, as in the dentist's chair, tension prevails and the pain can become what we expect it to be.

In somatoform pain disorder, the patient experiences pain, but the physician cannot explain the pain based on any test available or any disease that can be located. If a disorder is present, the pain is out of proportion to what one would ordinarily expect. I have been in the medical field long enough to see diseases remain undetected with the then-current diagnostic procedures, only to find that in later years, when new diagnostic tests became available, the diagnosis was more specific. For example, in the past many patients with pain running down the back of the leg were said to have negative findings when examined by an X-ray procedure called the spinal myelogram. Subsequently, when the same patients were examined with computed tomography (CT) scans, 30% of them were diagnosed as having herniated discs, which were the cause of the pain. As new procedures for diagnosing illness are discovered, the source of some pain syndromes will no doubt be uncovered.

No patient ever should be told by a friend, relative, or physician that the pain is in his or her head. Pain is subjective. It certainly can be aggravated by emotional distress, but the pain is real, and it should not be negated by others. It is well known that anxiety and depression can increase pain, but they are not the cause of pain. In fact, antidepressant medication has been helpful in reducing pain, even when the pain clearly is due to organic pathology such as cancer.

Because emotional factors can increase pain, in the course of psychotherapy, pain often will diminish if the emotional issues are handled appropriately by the patient. I have seen more than one patient deal with chronic pain in rather stoical ways with genuine acceptance of its chronic nature and a minimum of medication for the pain. In addition, I have seen patients respond favorably to audiotapes designed to relieve tension and reduce pain. Listening to the tapes enabled patients to be pain free for several hours at a time. A pain-free period, even for this amount of time each day, made the rest of the day more bearable.

The problem of pain is not well understood, but more research is being done by anesthesiologists, psychiatrists, psychologists, and others. I have seen some progress in the last 20 years, but we have a long way to go.

When a somatoform disorder cannot be categorized as one of the previously mentioned disorders, it is considered a somatoform disorder not otherwise specified.

Dissociative Disorders

The dissociative disorders are the subject of many novels, movies, and TV programs. The symptoms in this group of disorders are dramatic. Amnesia, dissociative identity disorder (multiple personality disorder), and fugue states are unusual and rare. Dissociative identity disorder is best exemplified by the movie *The Three Faces of Eve*, which is a true story. It is a disorder that I have never seen in a patient in more than 30 years of psychiatric practice. Some psychiatrists have seen a few cases; others claim to have seen many more.

I have treated several cases of amnesia, but these, too, are rare. Yet, the general public is familiar with these disorders via novels, movies, and TV, and the perception is that these ailments are common.

Dissociative Identity Disorder
(Multiple Personality Disorder)

In *The Three Faces of Eve*, Eve had three personalities: a prudish, conservative personality (Eve White); a sensual, seductive personality (Eve Black); and her "normal" social self (Eve). The changes in these personalities were rapid and unpredictable.

Although the patient with dissociative identity disorder may be aware of his or her various personalities, these are not contrived or acted out. They appear to be real, distinct personalities that are clearly differentiated from each other. Many psychiatrists now believe that patients with this disorder have been physically or sexually abused as young children. Although these patients may have been abused, I feel that more research is needed before this conclusion is scientifically valid.

Psychotherapy with these patients usually involves considerable time. It may require hypnosis, medication, and frequent sessions to get at the problems involved in this disorder. Although integration of the personalities is not always successful, it has been achieved in a number of cases. In the case of Eve, she married, raised several children, and reportedly fused her personalities successfully.

The book *Sybil*, by Flora Schreiber, is another true story of a young woman who had 16 personalities. (This book can still be obtained in paperback editions.)

Dissociative Amnesia

The most common form of dissociative amnesia has a short duration, lasting hours to days. There may be partial or complete amnesia for the experience. The following case example illustrates this disorder.

Case Example

John came to see me because of family problems. He was a conscientious father of five children. Because of a period of parental neglect in his childhood, John had decided to be a much better father to his children than his father had been to him. One day, while he drove through a severe thunderstorm with his family, John's car was disabled in a deserted area. John became alarmed and feared for the children's safety. However, he managed to call for help and finally negotiated the storm and got the family home safely. The next day, while at breakfast, he told his wife that he did not recall anything of the previous day. John had no memory of the storm or what he had done during that time. He had a complete amnesia for the stressful experience. To John, there was no greater threat than the possibility that his family would be harmed. It was so important that he was not able to contain the memory of the storm.

Amnestic events are not so rare. They may or may not require treatment. If the person has other problems, psychotherapy would certainly be recommended.

I have seen patients who have little recollection of the first part of their lives. One man could not remember any significant events of the first 20 years of his life. It may not be important to some individuals that they remember their past if their lives are going well. But if there are a number of other symptoms that interfere with their lives, they should seek treatment for these symptoms, as well as for the amnesia.

Dissociative Fugue

The onset of dissociative fugue tends to be sudden. It begins with a severe stress; this stress leads to an escape from conflict—a flight from the scene. The patient has no memory of the conflict or the reason for the flight. In addition, the patient also may adopt another identity. The new identity may have no relationship at all to his or her previous one. Again, this disorder makes great material for novels and movies. However, dissociative fugue is rare, and in my career, I have never seen a single case. Treatment of dissociative fugue usually requires traditional hypnosis or medical hypnosis to discover the person's true identity and bring him or her back to reality.

Depersonalization Disorder

Patients with depersonalization disorder speak of being out of touch with people: "I feel detached, as if I am not really present. Sometimes I feel as though I am looking down upon a scene in which I am a participant. At other times, I feel as though I am far away from where I am." Some individuals say they feel like they are in a dreamlike state or moving about with little feeling of control.

Depersonalization may occur briefly to anyone. Although the feelings of detachment are real, the person is in touch with reality and knows that the experiences are out of the ordinary.

Emotional conflict and a variety of stressors are responsible for depersonalization. It does not occur in any particular personality, nor is it associated with any disease. A patient who is neurotic can experience it, as well as someone who is in a psychotic state. Generally, it is not a disorder that a person would seek help for in the absence of other symptoms. More often, depersonalization is part of another set of symptoms. But to qualify as a complete disorder, it must be a persistent state that interferes with a person's overall functioning. Psychotherapy is the preferred method of treatment. Antianxiety medications sometimes can reduce the tension and stress in the patient and thereby indirectly decrease the depersonalization.

When the depersonalization does not fit the previously mentioned categories, it is classified as a dissociative disorder not otherwise specified.

What Can Families, Friends, and Caregivers Do?

Families, friends, and caregivers of those with neuroses can be understanding and sympathetic without being overly involved with the patients' anxiety disorders. For example, caregivers of patients with phobias or panic disorder should not always accommodate the patients and make everything pleasant by always avoiding the phobia or situation that induces panic. Accommodating patients only serves to increase their fear and does not help them push beyond their level of impaired functioning. In cases of agoraphobia, family members and friends should help the patients go out more or drive a little farther. They should encourage attacking the phobia rather than avoiding it. Caregivers can be understanding while being helpful in pushing patients ahead, much like a coach would do. The analogy of the Lamaze method comes to mind. Expectant mothers are supported and encouraged by the expectant fathers, who are called coaches. The mothers must do their work effectively to deliver the babies, but the coaches must be empathic and yet encourage the delivery to proceed.

Those supporting the patients also can be helpful in properly administering medication. It is sometimes necessary for family members to give medications to the patients, either because the patients take too much or, because of their anxiety disorder, they become confused and take their medications irregularly.

Encouraging proper nutrition without badgering patients is helpful. Equally important is insisting on proper exercise to reduce some of the anxiety.

There are many ways to be helpful. Timing is important. When patients are overwrought or excessively tired, it is not a good time for them to venture out and conquer a phobia. It is better to wait for the right opportunity when the situation is more relaxed. With proper psychiatric help and the involvement of family and friends, anxiety, so common to our generation, can be eliminated or severely curtailed. It is my contention that psychiatrists cannot work in isolation. They need all the help that they can get from their patients' relatives, friends, or other caregivers.

CHAPTER 8

ALCOHOLISM AND DRUG ABUSE

M y oldest brother's name was Andrew. He was born with a medical condition called torticollis—"wryneck." It was a disfiguring condition for which there was no cure at the time. Andrew had his moments when he could be kind and giving, but he mostly appeared lonely and disgruntled. I was the youngest of eight children, and from where I stood, I saw an unhappy man who was old enough to be my father, a man who had the misfortune of having alcoholism.

Andrew was the first to come to America—both a burden and an opportunity—with my father, while my mother and the younger children remained in Holland. The 15-year-old son and the 43-year-old father came seeking their fortune in the land of plenty. It was 4 years after World War I, and there were massive unemployment and poverty in Holland. One of my brothers remembers standing in a breadline with my mother. There were no jobs available in the local communities, and my father was forced to do something dramatic to support his family. He decided to go to America, with Andrew, as many others had done before. After 1 year of working in the United States, he saved and borrowed enough money to bring my mother and the rest of the children, ages 2 to 14 years old, to America. It was then a long sea voyage. The children were excited. They had heard about America with its wealth and cowboys. But the crossing was not pleasant. Seasickness made the trip difficult, but finally they arrived safely in New York Harbor. With the help of a Dutch family in New Jersey, they managed to secure temporary but crowded quarters. Gradually, my family gained a foothold in America. Although America had its problems, conditions were far better here than in Holland. After a while, my family felt at home with the immigrant Dutch community and the church that they found far away from the old country. I was born 7 years later.

Andrew became a house painter. He also began to drink heavily. I was not too aware of this as a young child, but when I became an adolescent, it became obvious to me. I remember the accidents he had with his car, his irritability, his arguments with the family, and his inability to work at times. But the most striking experience occurred one night just after I had returned from college. It was about midnight when I opened the door to our house and turned on the light. To my horror, Andrew was lying on the floor, a gash across his face. Apparently, he had attempted to put on the light and had fallen against the table. Having been unable to get up, he was asleep on the floor. I awakened him and helped him get to bed. I do not remember what happened the following day after this event. I am certain my mother suffered much grief seeing her firstborn son in this condition. All I can remember were failed attempts on the part of family members and elders of the church toward helping Andrew attain sobriety. At times, their intervention seemed to help, but mostly it did not matter. Andrew continued to live at home with my mother after all of us had gone our own way. He never married. He died of alcoholism at age 63.

We tried to help Andrew in our limited ways. But looking back on it, I think we offered more criticism than assistance. Only much later did it occur to me that he was more to be pitied than censured. Alcoholism was not considered a disease at the time. It was thought by most people to be a moral issue, a behavioral problem that one could change by simply making a decision to stop drinking. Somehow, the word about Alcoholics Anonymous (AA) had not reached us yet.

Much has changed since then. I have helped patients with alcoholism through periods of detoxification and followed them with outpatient care in conjunction with AA. Many have done well, are now sober, and are leading productive lives. Some never made it; they died from alcoholism and its physical consequences.

How Do I Know if Someone Is Alcohol Dependent?

Although it is a good question, people who have the disease seldom ask whether they have alcoholism. Rather, the question is raised by occasional drinkers who are preoccupied with their behavior. They are usually not alcohol dependent at all.

However, there are several ways to determine if someone is alcohol dependent. One standard is found in DSM-IV, which lists criteria for substance dependence. DSM-IV states that to have a diagnosis of alcohol or drug dependence, a person must manifest at least three of the following during a 12-month period:

(1) tolerance, as defined by either of the following:
   (a) a need for markedly increased amounts of the substance to achieve intoxication or desired effect
   (b) markedly diminished effect with continued use of the same amount of the substance
(2) withdrawal, as manifested by either of the following:
   (a) the characteristic withdrawal syndrome for the substance . . .
   (b) the same (or a closely related) substance is taken to relieve or avoid withdrawal symptoms
(3) the substance is often taken in larger amounts or over a longer period than was intended
(4) there is a persistent desire or unsuccessful efforts to cut down or control substance use
(5) a great deal of time is spent in activities necessary to obtain the substance (e.g., visiting multiple doctors or driving long distances), use the substance (e.g., chain-smoking), or recover from its effects
(6) important social, occupational, or recreational activities are given up or reduced because of substance use

(7) the substance use is continued despite knowledge of having a persistent or recurrent physical or psychological problem that is likely to have been caused or exacerbated by the substance (e.g., current cocaine use despite recognition of cocaine-induced depression, or continued drinking despite recognition that an ulcer was made worse by alcohol consumption)
(American Psychiatric Association 1994, p. 181)

It is amazing that persons with more than three of the above criteria will deny that they are alcohol or drug addicted. They will insist on their ability to control drinking and will minimize the effects it has had on work or family. They use the defense of denial so that they do not have to face their addiction.

How Common Is Alcoholism?

Years ago, alcoholism was regarded by most people as a moral issue. To put it simply, the attitude was, They're drunks. If they really wanted to stop, they could—it's just a bad habit. Many thought of alcoholism as a weakness of character. People of strong character just did not allow themselves to become alcohol dependent. Physicians and other health care workers had similar attitudes. Unfortunately, all too many of them also had serious problems with alcohol consumption. Alcoholism has no regard for a person's position, stature, wealth, or power. It cuts across social and ethnic lines. According to the Institute of Medicine, there are 13 million individuals who clearly or probably need treatment for alcohol use disorders. Of these 13 million, about two-thirds are men, and about one-third concurrently have more than one substance abuse disorder.

Alcoholism has long been the source of much trouble for humankind. It has contributed far more to premature deaths via accidents and disease than has drug addiction. The majority of families in this country are familiar with the tragic effect of alcoholism on one or more of their members. It costs the nation billions of dollars in health care spending as well as absenteeism from work.

One day, I was struck by the large number of patients I was

treating for alcoholism or who had alcoholic family members. As I looked over my office schedule, the number of patients with alcoholism or alcoholic family members amounted to about 50% of the patients whom I was seeing that week. And please note, I am in the general practice of psychiatry, and I do not specialize in alcoholism.

It is interesting that in some countries the incidence of alcoholism is less than it is here. Just why this difference exists is currently unclear. For example, in Italy and Japan the incidence is lower. Cultural differences probably play a part in accounting for this, but the exact reasons for the disparity are not known.

Drinking Habits

There are alcoholic individuals who drink an enormous amount of alcohol every day. Others have drinking bouts lasting for days or weeks, followed by periods of sobriety. Some drink all day long, whereas others drink mostly at night. There also are wide differences in the amount of alcohol that people can tolerate.

Persons who have a long history of heavy alcohol consumption have impaired liver function. They usually become intoxicated more quickly because the liver cannot detoxify the alcohol fast enough. There are individuals who acquire liver disease early, after only a relatively short time drinking, and others who drink excessively for an entire lifetime and never develop serious liver disease.

Reasons for Excessive Drinking

I have heard many rationalizations for heavy drinking, including "Everybody is doing it," "I need to have something in my hand in social situations," "It relaxes me," "It loosens me up," and "It helps my pain." I could go on. AA warns alcoholic persons to be aware of times when the need to drink is most prevalent by keeping in mind the acronym HALT. When individuals are *h*ungry, *a*ngry, *l*onely, and *t*ired, they most often have an increased need to drink.

Alcoholism begins early. There is a strong tendency for it to run in families. It is quite likely hereditary, although this has not been proven. According to the National Institute of Mental Health, if one parent has alcoholism, there is a 25% likelihood that the children will have alcoholism. If both parents are alcohol dependent, the percentage doubles to 50% for their children. These percentages are striking and are borne out in statistical studies of families of alcoholic patients.

Aside from the possibility of hereditary influences, there is a strong social force in our society that encourages drinking. This social force begins in elementary school and, through peer pressure, is strongly encouraged in high school and college. The pressure to drink that occurs in groups of adolescents is enormous. Through dramas and commercials, movies and TV also encourage drinking alcohol, clearly suggesting to various segments of society that drinking is "cool." All elements of society are affected, from tough street people to the middle class to the wealthy and sophisticated. Recently, however, there has been some effort by producers of daytime TV dramas to present less drinking and smoking.

Symptoms of anxiety and depression also lead to excessive drinking because many people discover that alcohol relieves their symptoms. For many others, alcohol does not relieve their symptoms. I know people who get sick from one drink. Others feel dizzy, feel nauseous, and have headaches after several drinks. Still others become sleepy when they drink more than a few ounces of alcohol. The likelihood that these people will become alcohol dependent is slim. Conversely, alcoholic individuals feel better when they drink. They do not feel the distressing symptoms that others do. Instead, they feel high and are relieved of their anxiety, depression, pain, or loneliness as they continue to drink. Many do not suffer much from hangovers and seem to tolerate copious amounts of alcohol, at least for a while. I am convinced that the relief of symptoms plays an important part in the development of alcoholism.

Forms of Alcoholism

Alcohol interferes with brain function in a variety of ways. This interference results in different manifestations of alcoholism.

In DSM-IV, disorders due to alcohol are classified as the following:

- Alcohol use disorders (alcohol dependence, alcohol abuse)
- Alcohol-induced disorders (intoxication; withdrawal; delirium due to intoxication or withdrawal; various dementias; psychoses with hallucinations or delusions; mood, anxiety, and sleep disorders; sexual dysfunction)

The six most common alcoholic illnesses are as follows:

1. *Alcoholic intoxication.* Alcoholic intoxication is the most familiar effect of excessive alcohol consumption. It results in poor coordination and interferes with abilities such as driving a car. Judgment becomes impaired, and sexual and aggressive impulses are altered. Under the influence of alcohol, individuals often change their behavior to such an extent that they perform antisocial acts that would not be possible for them while sober. There are responsible adults who get into fights in bars or beat their wives when intoxicated. When sober, they are alarmed at their behavior, although they do not necessarily stop drinking because of such actions.

2. *Alcohol withdrawal syndrome.* If the alcoholic individual suddenly stops drinking, he or she may experience nausea, vomiting, tremors, excessive perspiration, and rapid pulse. Mood alterations occur as well. Occasionally, convulsions and visual hallucinations are part of the syndrome. Assuming that the person does not drink during the withdrawal period, the symptoms may subside after 5–7 days.

3. *Alcohol withdrawal syndrome with delirium.* After discontinuing the consumption of alcohol, the alcoholic patient has alcohol withdrawal syndrome in addition to delirium. This disturbance consists of disorientation as to time and place, in-

creased visual hallucinations, and interference with recent memory and sleep. Tremors also are amplified, and convulsions are typical in untreated cases. This condition can lead to death in 20% of patients if not treated.

4. *Alcohol hallucinosis.* When chronic alcoholic patients stop drinking for a time, they may experience auditory hallucinations (hearing voices). These hallucinations may be similar to the hallucinations of the schizophrenic patient. The syndrome is not common. If severe, alcohol hallucinosis may require hospitalization. If the alcoholic patient remains sober, the condition will disappear in days. At times, it can last much longer.

5. *Alcohol amnestic syndrome (Wernicke-Korsakoff syndrome).* Chronic alcoholic patients may have short-term memory loss, confusion, and difficulty with balance and eye movements. With high doses of the vitamin thiamine, some of these symptoms may clear up. However, the confusion and memory loss may remain because of damage to brain cells by the chronic use of alcohol.

6. *Dementia associated with alcoholism.* With prolonged, excessive alcohol consumption, an individual may experience confusion, memory loss, and disorientation as to time and place. Later, some deterioration in personality functioning can occur, lasting for weeks or permanently.

The illnesses described above represent the effects of excessive use of alcohol on the brain. There are other equally dangerous diseases caused by alcohol. These diseases include neuropathies (nerve damage); bleeding of the stomach, esophagus, or intestinal tract; pancreatitis; and cirrhosis of the liver. In addition, fetal alcohol syndrome occurs if a baby's mother has been drinking excessively. Abnormalities in a newborn's weight and height are common. There also is a failure of the skull and brain to develop to normal size. Mental retardation can occur. Even small amounts of alcohol are suspected to cause defects in the developing fetus. As a result, expectant mothers are warned not to drink at all during pregnancy.

Treatment of alcoholism and drug abuse is discussed later in this chapter.

Drug Abuse

Describing all the drugs that are abused and the symptoms that result from their abuse is beyond the scope of this chapter. The drugs are all too familiar: marijuana, cocaine, heroin, and tobacco, to name a few.

Almost everyone knows of individuals who have had bouts with drug abuse. Rock singers, actors, and professional athletes discuss their drug abuse on talk shows or in books. It has become glamorized, and in the entertainment and sports world, it almost appears to be a rite of passage. But there is nothing glamorous about substance abuse. The biblical quote, Wine is a mocker, strong drink is raging: and whosoever is deceived thereby is not wise, applies equally to drug abuse. Its social and personal effects can be devastating, and for many, the effects have been deadly. DSM-IV criteria for substance dependence, listed earlier in this chapter, can be used to determine if someone is addicted to drugs.

I have talked with young people who were abusers of drugs before age 10 years. These children lived in the suburbs and were from middle- or upper middle–class families.

Case Example

Dora began using marijuana at age 9 years. Marijuana was followed by alcohol and later by other drugs, including LSD, cocaine, and various mixtures of drugs. When she was in her 20s, Dora said that she could not imagine going 1 day without being high on something. Although her statement sounded rather incredible to me at the time, I realized that the way she felt about drugs was not so different from alcoholic patients, who felt the same about alcohol. The only difference was that alcoholic patients usually denied their need for alcohol and stated that they were in control and could stop anytime.

I saw Dora for a few sessions, and it became obvious that she was caught up in a social scene of drug abuse from which she could not escape by herself. I could not help her in an outpatient office setting. She had to be taken out of this environment and placed in a rehabilitation clinic. After the first try at rehabilitation, Dora soon returned to her friends and the drug culture with which she was so familiar. We tried rehabilitation again, and it was more successful the second time. She received educational sessions on drug abuse and attended Narcotics Anonymous (NA) meetings regularly. On returning home, Dora continued to go to NA and got a job in an office where there was no drug use. She had to make a deliberate effort to sacrifice her relationships with her "druggie" friends for relationships with those who were not involved with drugs. Although this change was not without problems, Dora did manage to avoid her friends who used drugs.

Why do so many people, young and old, get caught in the drug net? Peer pressure, a sense of belonging, a need to experience something beyond the ordinary, the so-called mind-expanding sensations, and a million more personal reasons are all offered for drug use. For those who abuse alcohol or drugs, regardless of their reasons for using the substances, there is a common mental defense used. It is called denial. The importance of the substance to the individual and its harmful effects are denied. The drug abuser feels that he or she is in control and needs no help. This attitude prevails despite the reality of the situation—loss of a job, car accidents, and loss of relationships with family and friends. All kinds of rationalizations exist, such as "Everybody takes some drugs," "I can control it," "It's not a problem," and "I know people who take five times as much as I do." These and other comments are often heard among drug and alcohol abusers. There is the illusion of control that exists in the face of obvious loss of control. The degree to which the human mind can deny the reality of destructive forces has always amazed me.

Seldom does the addicted individual help himself or herself to sobriety. It usually takes dramatic crises and active treatment to turn around the lives of those addicted to alcohol and drugs. Most often, medical attention and group experiences with AA or NA are necessary to bring about this change.

Prevalence of Drug Abuse

The youth of today think that they invented drug abuse. It has been around for centuries. Drugs have been used in rituals by natives in many primitive countries. In Victorian times, cocaine was widely used. Since the early 1900s, the drugs of abuse mostly were alcohol, marijuana, and cocaine. Coca-Cola, for example, was an extract from the coca leaf and contained small amounts of cocaine. When its toxic effects became apparent, the active ingredients of cocaine were removed from the drink. During the depression years in the 1930s, there was little drug abuse except in the inner cities and especially among musicians and some artists.

One rainy fall day, I was on my way home to New Jersey from the medical school that I attended in New York City. It was Friday, and because of the rain, I was running to the subway along 110th Street. I was wearing a raincoat and was carrying an old suitcase. I suddenly noticed an old-model car traveling slowly beside me. One of the passengers yelled at me to stop. One look at him told me that I had better continue running. I maintained my pace, but he jumped out of the car and grabbed me. I tried to resist, but he quickly showed me the gun in his shoulder holster. I needed no more convincing. Now there were two men. They insisted that I open my suitcase. I thought to myself that these muggers were going to be very disappointed when they find out what's in there. I opened it and showed them my laundry and my books. I then asked why they had stopped me, and they explained that there had been some drug runners in the neighborhood and they were checking out suspects for drugs. They were plainclothes police. The year was 1950.

Then a revolution in substance abuse began. It started with Timothy Leary. He introduced mind-altering drugs to anyone who would listen. "Turn on, tune in, and drop out" became the slogan for disenchanted youth. This revolution led to Woodstock and other exhibitions of uninhibited sex, as well as alcohol and drug use. But drug abuse soon spread to younger people and to adults—middle-aged and even older adults. Soon, drugs became big business, and crime and drugs became partners in the inner cities and in the suburbs.

What has happened to drug abuse in the meantime? Since 1950, the use of street drugs has increased remarkably. A few years ago, the National Institute on Drug Abuse reported that after a rapid rise, the use of street drugs leveled off in the general population. In the case of marijuana, the incidence of its use among high school students declined. Cocaine use, which had become quite prevalent in the middle and upper middle class also declined somewhat. About 10% of high school seniors have used cocaine at least once. But after this reported decline in marijuana and cocaine abuse, drug abuse by children, adolescents, young adults, and older adults remains surprisingly high. A recent survey by the National Institute on Drug Abuse revealed that among 18,000 eighth graders, use of marijuana, cocaine, and LSD is again increasing.

Millions and perhaps billions of dollars are spent on drugs each year. Drug abuse also has increased the cost of health care because abusers often need emergency room and intensive care units in hospitals for treatment of their drug abuse.

Seldom do abusers of drugs and alcohol use only one substance. Rather, it is common for these individuals to use a number of substances in the search for the ultimate high. This condition is referred to as polysubstance abuse. Some of these people have a mental illness in addition to abusing drugs, which presents even greater problems to hospital personnel who must treat these dual problems.

Prescription Drugs

Years ago, medications prescribed by physicians were not highly regulated by the Food and Drug Administration. But there were relatively few drugs that were abused. Barbiturates and certain pain pills were the main addictive drugs available by prescription. More recently, there have been many tranquilizers and sleeping pills that have been introduced to the public. These have been appropriately used by many patients but grossly abused by others. Stimulants such as amphetamines and Ritalin (methylphenidate) have been strictly controlled for a number of years. Tranquilizers and hypnotics (sleeping pills) also have been controlled. Despite government controls, these drugs have gotten into the hands of drug dealers and have been sold on the black market. In addition, some physicians, nurses, and other medical personnel, by reason of their access to these drugs, have abused them to a large degree. Prescription drugs, as well as alcohol and marijuana, have been implicated as gateway drugs to further abuse of street drugs.

Prescription drugs can become the source of addiction themselves. Tranquilizers, sleeping pills, and pain pills are the drugs about which physicians are cautioned most often. In my experience, alcoholic patients and others who have a tendency toward addiction are the groups most likely to succumb to abuse of prescribed drugs. When patients are overly concerned about a tranquilizer being addicting, I seldom have to worry about these patients actually abusing the drug. But there are some people who inadvertently may become addicted because of lack of supervision or failure to get relief from their symptoms. Elderly patients with memory lapses are known to take more medication than is prescribed. It is the responsibility of the physician and the pharmacist to supervise proper medication use. It also helps if the family monitors a patient's drug use to prevent abuse. Of course, the patient must also accept some responsibility for drug use.

Personality and Drug Abuse

People with personality disorders have a greater than average tendency to abuse drugs. Yet, there is only one personality type that stands out as being more subject to drug abuse: the antisocial personality. Individuals with antisocial personality disorder have loose morals, weak consciences, and little regard for safety and health. They are more concerned with immediate gratification than are other people.

But aside from distinct personality types, there are at least two traits present in people who abuse drugs. The first trait is the need to experience unusual amounts of pleasure from outside sources. Whether this trait is because of hereditary or environmental factors, these individuals have difficulty resisting the pull to have these substances as part of their everyday life. I am convinced that drugs or alcohol provides an ongoing source of pleasure to abusers that is not possible with other people. For example, most individuals, when drinking excessively, develop headaches, intestinal difficulties, dizziness, or other symptoms that preclude further drinking. These symptoms do not readily affect alcoholic patients. The second trait found in substance abusers is that symptoms such as anxiety, depression, physical pain, or other distresses are relieved quickly with alcohol or drugs. In the experience of many substance abusers, ordinary medications do not give the relief that the abused substance provides. It is a question of symptom relief. Substance abusers feel more pleasure and symptom relief from drugs or alcohol than from any other source.

Treatment of Alcoholism and Drug Abuse

Years ago, when I first witnessed alcoholism in my family, the condition was thought to be a moral problem, not a disease. Since then, the medical profession has begun to accept alcoholism more as a medical problem. However, there is still a tendency for some physicians to deny that addiction to alcohol is a disease; to them, it is simply a matter of willpower. The same attitude prevails about drug abuse. I have heard physicians speak disparagingly about addicted persons. In one instance that I can recall, I saw a physician show little empathy and considerable rage toward an addicted patient when the patient had to be examined following an injury. In general, physicians' views on substance abuse have improved. I believe that most of the credit for this improvement should go first to AA. More recently, some physicians have come to specialize in the treatment of alcoholism and drug addiction. A few years ago, a group of psychiatrists formed an organization called the American Academy of Psychiatrists in Alcoholism and Addictions. At the national level, the Department of Health and Human Services has a subdivision called the Substance Abuse and Mental Health Services Administration.

When I started my psychiatric practice some 30 years ago, I was not familiar with some of the principles that are taught in AA. The idea that family members and friends can be *enablers* to alcoholic patients was not taught in medical school when I attended. Enablers allow alcoholic individuals to rebound from alcoholic bouts by being understanding and forgiving and by providing care, money, and whatever else enables these alcoholic persons to continue their addiction.

My elderly mother was an enabler without knowing it. She enabled out of compassion and concern for my alcoholic brother. Physicians also can become enablers. I am certain that I was an enabler in my early work with alcoholic patients before I became familiar with this concept. Early on, I prescribed tranquilizers to alcoholic patients to relieve their anxiety or morning "shakes." I thus enabled them to go on drinking. I have stopped this enabling, and I insist that patients attend AA in addition to psychotherapy. Some physicians feel it is useless to tell patients about their obvious alcoholism because they believe it would do no good. Such attitudes enable alcoholic individuals to continue drinking. Fortunately, younger physicians are being trained to understand the concept of enabling and the valuable work of AA.

Another AA concept is *codependency*. Early in my career, codependency was unknown to me, as it was developed in the last 15–20 years. Codependency refers to nonalcoholic individuals who become so enmeshed in their relationships with alcoholic persons that they become overly dependent on the alcoholic persons psychologically. Codependency can occur with anyone who is intimately involved with a deeply troubled individual. Thus, any relative, friend, or caregiver can become a codependent individual. Melody Beattie wrote an excellent self-help book on this subject. She is familiar with the concept of codependency because of personal experience. As a former alcohol and drug abuser, she knew people who were codependent with her. As a person in recovery who was counseling addicted individuals, she found herself codependent to such a degree that she was distressed and ineffective in her work. She studied the concept of codependency and wrote about it in her book, *Codependent No More*. After mentioning many definitions and examples of codependency, she offers a one-sentence definition: "A codependent person is one who has let another person's behavior affect him or her, and who is obsessed with controlling that person's behavior" (p. 31). This phenomenon is found among people involved with substance abusers, as well as individuals who have other physical and emotional illnesses. The codependent person leaves little time for his or her own needs. He or she is too busy trying to control the behavior of the other person. Codependency sometimes leads to tragic emotional consequences for the codependent person.

Enabling, codependency, and other concepts are discussed in meetings with families of alcoholic persons (Al-Anon) where relatives learn how to deal more effectively with their alcoholic family members. Other groups, such as Alateen and Adult Children of Alcoholics, also are helpful in learning about the ways of alcoholic individuals and how to deal with them. It is my opinion that AA is an important force in helping alcoholic individuals come to terms with their addiction and in keeping them sober. The same is true of NA. Some of the more senior members of AA become sponsors of new alcoholic members. These sponsors are only a telephone call away and help the alcohol or drug abuser with on-the-spot advice and counsel. Individuals who have survived the ravages of substance abuse know better than anyone how abuse can be rationalized and denied. They also know how to talk to members of groups such as AA and NA about avoiding the return to substance abuse. Untold numbers of substance abusers have been helped by these organizations. Although medical treatments are often necessary for detoxification and to begin rehabilitation, the long-range commitment to sobriety by substance abusers is best kept with the strong support of these self-help groups. Then, if psychiatric illnesses exist despite sobriety, these can be treated in combination with AA, NA, or other group meetings as needed.

AA and NA demand honesty of their members in confronting the lack of power over the abused substance. As part of the 12 steps toward sobriety, members are asked to seek help from a higher power, make amends with whomever they have offended while under the influence of abusive substances, and correct behavior that is destructive to their relationships with others. In open and closed meetings, members face their denial and cope with the reality of their addiction.

Substance abuse can occur along with serious depression, schizophrenia, or any other psychiatric disorder. When alcohol or drug abuse is present in a patient who also has a psychiatric disorder, it is referred to as a mental illness and chemical abuse grouping or a *dual diagnosis*. Many hospitals have beds set aside for patients with a dual diagnosis. The decision to treat one disease first depends on which is the most urgent, acute, or life threatening. For example, if someone has schizophrenia and simultaneously has delirium tremens due to sudden withdrawal from alcohol, the physician treats the delirium tremens first because this condition is potentially lethal and takes only days to control. Once physically stable, the patient is treated for the schizophrenia. It is common to see a patient who has a chemical abuse problem and depression. Sometimes the drug or alcohol abuse itself can be the cause of the depression. If so, the physician first concentrates on detoxifying the patient of the abused substance. Then, if the depression remains, appropriate antidepressants are used for dealing with the depression.

Thus, the psychiatrist must be aware that more than one illness may be present at the same time. On occasion, some patients hide the fact that they are drinking alcohol or are taking a mind-altering drug. Hiding their habit makes treatment difficult and may prolong the process of care.

What Can Families, Friends, and Caregivers Do?

One of the main problems encountered by families, friends, and caregivers of substance abusers is the defense of denial. Just as the abusers deny their abuse, those around substance abusers also deny that the problem is as severe as it is. The feelings of concerned people who are trying to help alcohol or drug abusers are so strong that they are all too ready to forgive the abuse and start over again, thereby enabling the substance abusers to continue their abuse. A thorough understanding of this interaction is important so that family members, friends, and caregivers really can be helpful. Often, it is necessary to say no to substance abusers when they ask for money, support, and even housing. Any caregiver should think carefully about the concept of codependency.

Perhaps the most difficult part of really helping substance abusers is allowing them to "hit bottom," the expression used in AA. This expression refers to abusers reaching the lowest level of their dysfunction, the point where they realize that they no longer are able to help themselves. Only when abusers hit bottom can they truly reach out for help to a higher power, as suggested by AA. As long as substance abusers deny their need for help and believe that they can do it on their own, they are likely to fail. Although I have seen a few patients obtain sobriety by their own means, most have failed. Sobriety is difficult to achieve without the help of self-help groups. I have been extremely grateful to AA and similar groups for creating a lifesaving and life-giving opportunity for substance abusers. It has changed many individuals and allowed them to truly live again.

Caregivers must not be overly sympathetic to substance abusers. They must genuinely help abusers to overcome their addiction and not enable abusers to continue their addiction. A tough-love approach is necessary in dealing with substance abusers. Caregivers should not try to do it all themselves. Rehabilitation of the substance abusers may be necessary, followed by their regular attendance at AA or NA meetings.

CHAPTER 9

SEXUAL PROBLEMS IN OUR CULTURE

How could a couple be married for 15 years and never have sexual contact? Why does a man desire to expose himself to young women in public? Why do men rape and kill? Why is there so much cruel and sadistic sexual behavior? Why are we so curious about sex? The answers to these questions are not readily available to us as yet, and the mystery surrounding sexuality is still greater than our knowledge about the subject. But some things are known.

Along with wealth and power, sex is among the most highly talked about subjects in our culture. It is the theme of books, movies, and plays and the fixation of magazine and newspaper articles. There is hardly a movie produced or a novel written that does not involve romantic love stories, sexual experimentation, or prurient fantasies of sexual intimacies. Sex is a topic that is at once full of delight, fear, torment, and perplexity.

Sexual needs are obsessively driven in some individuals; in others, the needs are more tempered. In some others, the needs are so strong that judgment is often suspended for the sake of satisfying lustful intent. To me, it is surprising how often people disregard the obvious threats to life and health by ignoring the known infectious hazards such as venereal diseases and especially exposure to acquired immunodeficiency syndrome (AIDS).

In humans, sexual needs are intimately connected with psychological needs. These psychological needs may be normal, ordinary needs such as the desire for intimacy and the elevation of self-esteem. The mental aspects of sexuality cannot be divorced from the sexual act, even in its simplest form.

Although it would be hard to prove, the sexual acts between animals probably contain mental components as well. The mating rituals of animals and birds attest to the fact that sexual expression is not simply a matter of copulation. The required prelude, when successfully acted out in mating rituals, allows the physical act of sex to happen. Only in the human imagination can the sexual act take on painful, cruel, grim, and sometimes deadly consequences. But even in these extreme instances, certain psychological needs are met—although they may be pathological needs.

In normal human development, there are at least two needs that are apparent in the young person after puberty. There is a strongly felt physical need—a sexual lust for contact with another human being—and a simultaneous need for closeness and intimacy. Some individuals have sexual desires that are not accompanied by feelings of psychological intimacy. These persons may be limited to sex with prostitutes or partners who also are not interested in furthering intimacy of any kind. Such individuals have failed to integrate lustful and intimacy needs. The opposite condition also may occur. Some persons cannot feel lustful toward those whom they love. Their need for intimacy is overwhelming, and the fantasy of the loved one is overly idealized. They may be very much "in love," but they are not able to have any sexual feelings for the other person.

Some years ago, I met a married couple at a mental health clinic. Although initially attracted to each other for physical and emotional reasons, they had never experienced sexual intercourse during the 15 years of their marriage. The husband was suffering from a primary impotency. His wife had sexual needs, but over the years, she had suppressed them to the extent that she no longer felt any physical desire to have sex. Meanwhile, the marriage had met the emotional needs of the couple to the extent that satisfied both of them. They planned to continue their relationship, stating that they had remained in love and saw no reason to break up the marriage.

To have a full and satisfying relationship, a couple should be able to feel, appreciate, and fulfill both lust and intimacy needs. At times, the lust may predominate, and at other times, the need for intimacy may be more obvious. Failure to integrate these two needs may result in a poor relationship. When there is a failure to integrate needs in marriage, the relationship can be quite strained. I have seen marriages in which the husband is preoccupied with obtaining sexual gratification and the wife is more interested in being emotionally intimate. In these situations, any attempt on the part of the wife to be affectionate is immediately perceived by the husband as a request for sexual contact, thus creating considerable stress.

There is another phenomenon that is common to humans. Men appear to be more compulsive about their sexual needs, whereas women are less compulsive and more influenced by other concerns. The study of sexual desires in men shows that their needs are compulsively driven. Compulsions are evident in the paraphilias, such as exhibitionism, fetishism, sadism, and rape. In sexual compulsions, the need is so strong that despite cultural restrictions and legal punishments, the acts are carried out anyway. Among women, compulsive sexual acts are far less common, although it could be argued that they occur in more subdued forms. For example, women can exhibit their sexuality by dressing provocatively without breaking the law.

By contrast, women are more concerned about nest building and the security of family life. These concerns may be cultural to some extent, but they appear to be present in all civilizations. Nest building and security are probably related to childbirth and child rearing. The man's expectation that his sexual needs be met on a regular basis does not necessarily coincide with the woman's need for nest building and security. In some marriages, these needs cause severe conflict. Considerable understanding is required of the marriage partners in order to resolve their various needs.

Changes Since the Sexual Revolution

Has the increase in sexual freedom changed society for the better? Freud spoke of the effects of sexual restraints on society. He believed that the repression of sexual needs and aggression was responsible for the anxiety disorders that he witnessed during the late 1800s. If this were true, the sexual freedom and increased aggression now present in Western countries should have brought about less anxiety and neurosis. This decrease has not occurred. In fact, it could be argued that anxiety has actually increased in recent years despite the sexual permissiveness that has permeated society.

What has resulted from our sexual freedom? From where I sit in the consultation room, I have observed that the lowering of inhibitions about sexuality has reduced some problems and brought about others. I am not at all certain that we have gained anything by the liberation of our sexual habits. I do not find many people more content with their sexual lives now than before the sexual revolution. I do see a great deal of confusion about sexual roles. On some college campuses, for example, first-year female students are confronted by other women and asked to declare their sexual preference. They are, in effect, pressured to state whether they are lesbian, heterosexual, or bisexual. This kind of pressure on a young woman is difficult, and for some, it can lead to greater anxiety about sex and confusion about sexual orientation.

With its emphasis on sexual freedom, this culture has made many young people doubt their sexual adequacy. Recently, there has been a notable increase in potency problems in men, as women have become more demanding of men for sexual satisfaction. It is my conclusion that the change in the sexual mores in our country has not solved the problems of sexuality; rather, the problems have been altered. The difficulties seen now are different and possibly harder to resolve because of the greater expectations for sexual fulfillment. There are other changes as well. When I went to medical school and worked in the urban environment, I witnessed common-law marriages. At that time, virtually no couple in the suburbs lived together outside of marriage. Today, many couples try living together to see if they are compatible. It has surprised me that many of these couples do not remain together for long if they choose marriage. Why? As far as I am aware, no studies have been done to answer this question. My guess is that living together is a different experience from that of marriage. The latter requires a whole "package" of common responsibility and commitment that is not found in the temporary arrangement of the couple living with each other. Marriage involves a sharing of goals and the molding of a family unit that is absent in the experimental day-to-day living arrangement of the unmarried modern couple. Young adults with whom I have spoken have described this situation and its lack of commitment as "playing house." In contrast, the institution of marriage requires attention to the mutual solution of life's problems, the sharing of life's joys, and the mature love, support, and comfort of a long-term relationship.

For all its delight and excitement, the sexual experience in humans is not without its aberrations and problems. Unfortunately, there are many. The following discussions are a summary of the disorders of sexuality found in our culture.

Sexual Disorders

The problems in sexuality can be categorized as follows:

- Gender identity disorders
- Paraphilias
- Sexual dysfunctions

There are various manifestations of the sexual disorders. Case examples as seen in the practice of psychiatry illustrate these manifestations.

Gender Identity Disorders

There are two aspects to gender identity. The first is psychological. It consists of the awareness of being male or female and includes some acceptance of this as a fact of life. The second aspect of gender identity is biological. It is a recognition that one possesses physical sexual characteristics of the male or the female. On occasion, a person does not accept his or her sexuality. Thus, a young man wishes to be a woman, or a young woman wants to live her life as a man. This rare disorder is called *transsexualism*. It occurs more often in males than females.

Case Example

I was asked to consult with a 14-year-old girl in my office. Her name was Jackie. She had told everyone that she had no intention of remaining a girl. She already had done everything she could to look like a boy, such as wearing male clothing, wearing her hair like a boy, and using a tight bra to hide her developing breasts. In her memory of early childhood, she had never felt like a girl in any way. She had always thought of herself as a boy named Jack. Even at her young age, she had contacted clinics in California to inquire about a sex change operation, which she had every intention of obtaining as soon as she was legally and financially able. Jackie recognized her female biological self, but her gender identity was clearly male. When I saw Jackie, I felt her orientation was so fixed that changing the psychological state of this young girl would have been an impossible task.

Just how such a situation comes about is not exactly known, although there are recorded cases in which a parent dressed and conditioned the child to be the opposite sex from infancy. If discovered early enough, this type of conditioning can be reversed. Much research is needed to figure out the origin of gender disturbances of this kind.

What factors affect sexual identity? There are at least three that have been confirmed through research:

1. Genetic factors become manifest in the fetus as early as the sixth week of pregnancy.
2. Characteristics such as physique, size, shape, facial features, and other physical traits play a part in determining gender identity.
3. A child's interactions with his or her parents, siblings, peers, and teachers, as well as the child's particular culture, all com-

bine to influence his or her gender identity. For example, if a young male toddler were dressed and treated like a girl by his mother, who wanted the child to be female, it certainly could cause psychologically based gender confusion in the child. But it would not necessarily make that child want to become a girl.

One of the problems of gender identity disorders is that these disorders are not brought to the psychiatrist until the child is well developed and has reached adolescence. Before this time, most children would not have made their confusion about gender identity known. However, if a gender disorder is discovered early enough and there is psychotherapeutic intervention, it is possible that the child's gender disorder could be changed. But once a child reaches adolescence, these gender disorders are extremely difficult to change. Regardless of the external sexual characteristics, the psychological set is hard to alter. As illustrated in the previous case example, Jackie had no desire to change.

Paraphilias

A *paraphilia* is a compulsive desire to have sexual fantasies and experiences that are not commonly practiced in the general population. The older term for paraphilias was *perversions*. The desires are felt as uncontrollable urges to the person involved. They are pleasurable and exciting but often are followed by guilt, remorse, and emotional conflict. Because most of the paraphilias are against the law in most states, legal problems are not uncommon for those who have these disorders.

The three main types of paraphilias are as follows:

1. Extreme sexual attraction to children or other persons who do not wish to engage in sexual acts.
2. Extreme attraction to objects belonging to another person, usually of the opposite sex. An example is a man who has a fetish about women's shoes.
3. An extreme desire to inflict pain or discomfort on others or oneself for the purpose of experiencing sexual excitement. In-

dividuals who are paraphilic have fantasies about sex and often act these out in reality, thus creating considerable sexual excitement and orgasm. If a person has an occasional paraphilic fantasy, it is not considered to be a paraphilic disorder. The fantasy has to be chronic, persistent, compulsive, and acted upon often to be considered a disorder.

Persons who have paraphilias often feel guilty about their preoccupations and acts. These individuals sometimes seek out the help of professionals to deal with their problems. Others, who feel little guilt, are only brought to psychiatrists or other professionals because of legal complications after breaking the law. Individuals in the latter group need to attend institutional programs for sexual offenders. Outpatient treatment for severe sexual offenders is not helpful, but those individuals who have had a late onset of sexual deviations or have committed only one or two offenses can often be helped by outpatient treatment.

Why do we seldom hear about female sexual offenders? Paraphilias appear to be more common among men although recently, women have been implicated for sex offenses, particularly in nurseries and child care centers. A book by Louise J. Kaplan, *Temptations of Emma Bovary*, suggests that women act out their deviant sexual disturbances by other means. She specifically cites symptoms such as eating disorders, shoplifting, and provocative dressing, which is still in the range of the socially acceptable. A good example of acting out a sexual disturbance is anorexia. Being extremely thin may be a young woman's way of denying her sexuality and trying to remain a child. Alternately, she can be on constant exhibition to others by her emaciated appearance and thus evoke sympathy and concern.

In DSM-IV, a number of paraphilias are described.

Pedophilia.   Pedophilia is a compulsive urge to contact children for the purpose of sexual arousal and satisfaction. The children, by definition, have not as yet reached puberty and must be at least 10 years younger than the other person involved.

I have treated adults who, as children, have been molested by parents, stepparents, grandparents, siblings, other relatives, neighbors, or friends. These early experiences of sexual abuse in childhood often create fear, guilt, and low self-esteem in the affected children. Persons who become pedophilic often have been molested in their own childhood. For reasons that are not clear, they have a need to repeat the experience when they, themselves, are older. These individuals usually have poor adult sexual relationships and feel extremely insecure. They have difficulty approaching an adult and working out a mutually consenting sexual relationship. By contrast, with children, they feel they can control the situation and dominate the children. Furthermore, children are easily plied with toys, candy, and threats, thus increasing the control over the children by individuals with pedophilia.

The aberrant behavior of those who have pedophilia can temporarily increase their self-esteem. The urge to commit pedophilic acts is so strong that they occur despite the obvious legal threats and the possibility of long jail sentences.

The effect of sexual abuse on the developing child is variable and depends on many factors. First of all, the age of the child is important. If the abuse occurs before the age of 2 years, there is little evidence that the child will remember the experience. At that age, it would be impossible to know how it would affect the child. As the child grows older and is better able to remember the abuse, the danger of psychological trauma increases. But there are also other factors. If the abuser is brutal, sadistic, cruel, and threatening, it creates a far worse trauma than if the abuser is gentle and convincing. The duration and frequency of the abuse also are important (one or two events versus many contacts over a long period of time). In addition, if the child reports the abuse to one of his or her parents, how the parent receives and reacts to the news is important. Some parents do not believe the child; others react with violent feelings. If the abuse occurs during adolescence, there is the additional factor of guilt. The adult who recalls adolescent sexual abuse is often haunted with doubt about his or her participation. Questions arise as to what degree the abused person willingly cooperated or physically or emotionally enjoyed the experience.

Another puzzling aspect of sexual abuse is that a number of people who were abused as children do not seem to be badly scarred as a result of the abuse. I have had patients tell me that they were abused when young; they reported it as part of their history. These patients came to see me for completely different reasons, not because of the sexual abuse. When asked about the impact of the abuse on their lives, these individuals denied that it had any major effect. How prevalent this phenomenon is, I do not know.

Recently, there has been a surge of newspaper articles about the increase in pedophilia. Although research on this topic is not solid, there does seem to be an actual increase in pedophilia—at least much more is being reported to the authorities. Some workers in this field believe that the number of pedophilic individuals in the general population is far more than is currently reported. Others, such as Dr. Richard Gardner, a child psychiatrist at the Columbia University College of Physicians and Surgeons in New York, do not agree. In *True and False Accusations of Child Abuse,* Gardner maintains that the incidence of child abuse within families is high and probably true when reported. But he feels that the incidence of abuse of children in nurseries and preschool settings is overestimated to the point of hysteria. He bases this opinion on his work as a child psychiatrist as well as much legal work concerning child abuse. He believes that children are impressionable and are easily led to make statements about sexual abuse by those who test the children and ask provocative questions. He compares the hunt for pedophilic individuals to the Salem witch trials. My own impression is that there is too much enthusiasm for finding the "culprit" at this time. I basically agree with Dr. Gardner, although it will take a while before the incidence of pedophilia is calculated with some degree of accuracy.

In *Suggestions of Abuse,* experimental work done by Dr. Stephen Ceci of Cornell University is described. Ceci's work illustrates how memory can be influenced greatly by suggestion. He reports that when young children are asked many questions about a given event, they tend to make up stories that are known to be false. His findings indicate that the suggestibility of young children seriously distorts their memories of events.

As families become less stable and both parents are in the work force, the need for day care or nursery school increases. As these social changes occur, it is likely that the incidence of pedophilia will increase. Regardless of how much competent adult supervision there is, pedophilia will not be eliminated completely. One of the reasons for this is the obvious compulsive need of the pedophilic individual to perform acts of abuse on children. Any compulsive act that is associated with pleasure is hard to change. Most individuals with pedophilia are referred to psychiatrists by the court only after the discovery of child abuse. I have only had one person who came to me for treatment of pedophilia in the absence of legal threats forcing him to do so.

Even with residential treatment for sexual abusers, the success rate for pedophilia is low. It is my opinion that a substantial number of pedophilic individuals do stop their abuse when the abused child moves out of the home. The convenience and familiarity of the home are often conducive to acting out pedophilic urges; the person with these desires may not dare to seek out a child in the neighborhood or local school.

Mental health professionals have a long way to go in understanding the reasons behind pedophilic behavior.

Fetishism.   Fetishism involves intense sexual desires and fantasies with the use of female clothing. Shoes, underwear, wigs, or other female garments may be used for the purpose of sexual stimulation. Little is known about the cause of fetishism.

Transvestic fetishism.   Transvestic fetishism is the desire for a man to wear female clothing and dress up to appear like a woman for the purpose of sexual excitement or fantasy. Cross-dressing is often associated with depression, guilt feelings, or anxiety. It begins as an act done in private but may evolve into a public act. It may be partial, as with a man wearing female underwear covered by his trousers, or it may be complete, as with a man dressing to appear as a woman. If the man is married, it can cause considerable stress in the marriage. Sometimes marriage partners are not upset by the transvestite behavior and use it as part of their sexual fantasy.

Exhibitionism.   Exhibitionism is the act of exposing the genitals to unsuspecting persons, usually women. It occurs almost entirely in men. The purpose of the exhibition is to alarm a woman and to see her reaction to the exposure. Although women often are alarmed and frightened by such men, these men are seldom dangerous. I have never encountered an exhibitionist who was also a rapist. Men who exhibit themselves are usually passive and are timid about forming relationships with women. They have a strong need to demonstrate their sexuality blatantly. Exhibitionists seldom seek help unless they are apprehended by the police. They seem to have considerable denial of their aberrant behavior.

Case Example

One day I talked with Joe in my office. He had been told by his lawyer that he had to see a psychiatrist about recent charges of exhibitionism. He was a slender, passive man who made it clear that he had come to my office reluctantly. But as we talked, he seemed to derive some relief from finally telling someone about his long-standing desire to exhibit himself. Although he had been apprehended only once, he confessed to numerous sexual exposures to young women. Joe was married and had two children. He and his wife communicated poorly and had infrequent sexual encounters. He also reported problems with his underlings in his work as an office manager. He had a low self-esteem that had bothered him for years. Joe had little experience with dating as a young man, and his wife was the first and only woman with whom he had had sex. Before his marriage, Joe did not have the courage to ask anyone else out on a date. His wife had been kind to him and mildly aggressive. Only with someone like her was he able to develop a relationship beyond mere friendship.

Joe's problems centered around his passivity and fears of rejection. Surprisingly, he became a motivated patient. With a desire to change and a wish to improve his marriage, he was able to control his exhibitionist tendencies successfully. In treatment, it is helpful to have the married couple come to therapy for joint counseling. Exhibitionism is more responsive to outpatient psychotherapy than are the other paraphilias.

Sexual sadism.   Sexual sadism consists of recurrent sexual fantasies and acts in which other persons are psychologically and/or physically abused. It involves inflicting pain for the purpose of sexual arousal. The term *sadism* is taken from the writings of the Marquis de Sade, who was notorious for sexual abuse of women.

How does sadism develop in humans? Oddly enough, this sexual disorder does not seem to be present in animals. One precondition for the occurrence of sadism is a history of violence in the families of affected persons. Sadistic individuals seem to have the need to repeat what they have experienced in their childhood. Somehow the sexual urge is associated with the desire to inflict pain. Often, there is a need to control the other person through the sexual encounter. It is based on the unconscious fear of being controlled by the other person as actually may have happened in childhood. The experience of being the controlling one who inflicts pain is sexually stimulating to the sadist.

Persons with sexual sadism rarely come to the attention of psychiatrists unless they are apprehended for legal reasons for abusing others.

Sexual masochism.   Sexual masochism is the opposite of sadism. The masochistic person enjoys associating the sexual act with pain or fantasies about pain. Sexual masochism also may involve being physically restrained, such as being tied or chained to a bed.

How or why these urges occur is not entirely clear. Persons who enjoy sexual masochism usually have a history of abuse in their childhood. Linking pain and sexual enjoyment can sometimes be recalled by individuals with this disorder. However, it is unusual for people who are sexual masochists to come to a psychiatrist for treatment because there is little need to change what they enjoy.

The terms *sadism* and *masochism* have become common in our literature, as well as in everyday usage. When individuals are described as sadistic, the word may mean that they are uncaring of others, they enjoy making others feel uncomfortable, they are excessively critical, they embarrass people, and generally, they have a mean streak. Similarly, when we speak of persons as masochistic, we mean that they are often taken advantage of, they do not assert themselves enough, and they frequently put themselves at the mercy of others. These terms do not refer to sexual behavior; rather, they refer to ingrained personality traits that are characteristic of a person. Such traits should not be confused with the paraphilias sexual sadism and sexual masochism.

Voyeurism.   Voyeurism is the desire to be sexually stimulated by viewing someone who is undressing, naked, or involved in sexual acts. Voyeurs do not want to be seen by those whom they are viewing. Voyeurism is usually done with simultaneous masturbation. One or two episodes of voyeurism by an adolescent does not make the person a voyeur. It must be present for at least 6 months to qualify as voyeurism.

I do not know if the incidence of voyeurism has decreased or not in recent years. I do know that when I was first in the practice of psychiatry 30 years ago, I periodically would get referrals from attorneys concerning voyeurs. In recent years, I have not had a single referral for voyeurism. I have wondered about this, and I have concluded that anyone who has a compulsion to view nude persons or sexual acts can easily satisfy this prurient interest by purchasing pornographic videotapes. By doing so, the individual can avoid being discovered and avoid subsequent legal problems.

Frotteurism.   Frotteurism is a paraphilia in which a man seeks sexual gratification by rubbing his penis against a woman's buttocks in crowded public places such as on buses, on subways, and in elevators. The incidence of this paraphilia is low. I have never known of a person to come for treatment for this disorder unless remanded to do so by the court.

Paraphilia not otherwise specified.   Disorders in the not otherwise specified category are rare and not generally seen by psychiatrists. The only one that is more common and may be seen by mental health professionals is telephone scatologia (preoccupation with obscene telephone calls). Such calls are illegal and are subject to prosecution. The other paraphilias are not likely to come to the attention of the authorities. These paraphilias are coprophilia (preoccupation with feces), urophilia (preoccupation with urine), mysophilia (preoccupation with unclean surroundings), and zoophilia (preoccupation with animals) and are all associated with sexual activities. Zoophilia, for example, is a strong urge to use animals for sexual gratification. This urge may occur as a transient phenomenon in children who are sexually attracted to farm animals or pets. If the urge persists into adulthood and becomes a dominant sexual desire, it then is a paraphilia. Although rarely seen by psychiatrists, zoophilia is probably more common than believed. The most bizarre form of paraphilia is necrophilia—sexual fantasies of or sexual contact with a dead person. As with many other paraphilias, persons who have these preoccupations do not seek psychiatric help.

Sexual Dysfunctions

The human sexual apparatus is complicated enough when we consider the anatomy, blood supply, nerve fibers, and normal physiology of the sexual act. But when the emotional factors that make up sexuality in humans are added to the equation, it is surprising that there are not more problems with sexuality than exist. The main sexual dysfunctions are reviewed in the following discussions.

Sexual Desire Disorders

Hypoactive sexual desire disorder.   An individual with hypoactive sexual desire has infrequent sexual fantasies and little or no desire for sexual activity of any kind. This disorder may occur for physical or emotional reasons. Common diseases that are associated with decreased sexual desire are diabetes, cardiac disease, and neurological disorders. Excessive alcohol and drug use and certain prescribed drugs, especially antihypertension medication, can cause this problem as well.

Although decreased sexual drive is common in old age, this condition may occur at any age after puberty. It is more common among women than men.

Emotional reasons for decreased sexual interest are many. Hostility and anger between partners are common causes. Traumas to one or the other partner, physical disabilities, or surgical procedures may turn off a partner to sexual activity. A depressed mood and clinical depression, whether mild, moderate, or severe, are especially corrosive to sexual desire. Loss of a marital partner can cause sexual disinterest in the survivor. Loss of finances or any other loss that causes depression can be devastating to sexual desire.

Sexual aversion disorder.   Sexual aversion disorder can be seen as a strong negative reaction to anything sexual or as an actual phobia toward sexual thoughts or acts. Physical symptoms may be associated with this disorder. Usually, there is a history of sexual abuse, excessive scolding, and punishment for sexual explorations of childhood with subsequent guilt about sex. This disorder is found more often in women.

Sexual Arousal Disorders

There are two disorders in this category: 1) female sexual arousal disorder and 2) male erectile disorder. By definition, in both of these conditions, sexual desire is present, but there are problems in sexual arousal and therefore performance.

Female sexual arousal disorder.   In female sexual arousal disorder, a woman feels sexual desires but is not able to reach a state of sexual excitement. The normal physiological responses such as vaginal lubrication do not occur. This condition used to be called sexual frigidity.

In women, organic problems such as hypothyroidism, hormonal variations, endocrine disorders, infections, diabetes, and neurological disorders can interfere with sexual feelings and sexual fulfillment. If a woman can achieve sexual excitement and orgasm through masturbation and not via intercourse, the problem is not usually due to physical causes.

Male erectile disorder.   In male erectile disorder, the man is not able to obtain an erection, has a partial erection, or is not able to maintain an erection long enough to complete the sexual act. It is estimated that about 10%–20% of males have erectile problems at some time. About 8% of young adult males are impotent and not able to have an erection at all.

What causes this disorder in men? Organic reasons for impotence are circulatory, neurological, or endocrine problems, such as diabetes. There are a variety of tests that can rule out these organic causes of impotence. If they prove to be negative, then the problem is assumed to be psychological. If a man has early morning erections and is able to reach a full erection with masturbation, it generally is a sign that the potency problem has a psychological base rather than an organic cause.

Anxiety is the most common psychological reason for failure to perform sexually. Depression, fatigue, pain, preoccupations, and distractions also are known to interfere with sexual fulfillment. When such problems exist, psychotherapy or specific sex therapy is helpful in alleviating the condition.

Usually, the ability to perform sexually continues through age 70 years and older. Many persons who are in their 80s have an active sexual life, although most individuals older than age 80 are not sexually active.

Orgasmic Disorders

Female orgasmic disorder.   About 5% of the female population have anorgasmia. With this disorder, a woman is not able to experience orgasm whether by masturbation or with sexual intercourse. About 30% of women have difficulty obtaining an orgasm, although they are not completely anorgasmic. This disorder may be due to fear of pregnancy, a history of sexual abuse in childhood, guilt feelings, preoccupation with responsibilities, or other psychological factors.

Male orgasmic disorder.   In about 5% of males who are physically well, there is an inability to experience ejaculation during intercourse. However, these individuals may be able to have an ejaculation with masturbation. A number of organic causes are responsible for orgasmic disorders in males. Among them are prostate disease, neurological disorders such as Parkinson's disease, and drug reactions (antihypertensive drugs and tranquilizers).

Premature ejaculation.   When a man ejaculates before or soon after he enters his partner's vagina, he has premature ejaculation. The

WHAT EVERY PATIENT, FAMILY, FRIEND, AND
156   CAREGIVER NEEDS TO KNOW ABOUT PSYCHIATRY

disorder is usually caused by anxiety about performance, and it is a common reason for seeking help from a psychiatrist. About 30%–40% of men who complain of sexual problems seek help for premature ejaculation. It is often caused by early traumatic experiences associated with guilt, secrecy, and punishment.

Sexual Pain Disorders

Dyspareunia.   Dyspareunia is the experience of pain before, during, or after intercourse. It can occur in both men and women but is much more common in women. Dyspareunia may be due to stress or organic diseases. In women, common causes are infection, inflammation, and tumors.

Vaginismus.   Vaginismus is a constriction of the outer one-third of the vagina, which makes intercourse difficult or impossible. The disorder can be brought on by fear or a history of rape or other sexual trauma. Pain, religious preoccupations, guilt, and fear of pregnancy are also causes.

In addition to the previously mentioned sexual disorders, DSM-IV includes two other types of sexual disorders: sexual dysfunction due to a general medical condition and substance-induced sexual dysfunction.

Treatment of Sexual Disorders

As noted earlier in this chapter, most paraphilias are not treatable in the general psychiatrist's office. Few persons with pedophilia, exhibitionism, or any other paraphilia ever go to a psychiatrist on their own for help. The compulsive and pleasurable nature of these disorders produces little desire for treatment of the conditions. Most of the patients with these problems come for treatment because they have been ordered to do so by the court, following apprehension for paraphilic behavior. Most patients with paraphilias are placed in special settings reserved for treatment of these difficult problems.

Reports released from these institutions show some success, but many of these patients repeat the problem and require further help. Months and years of treatment often are necessary. In a number of states in this country, sexual offenders are placed in jail rather than in treatment facilities.

An exception to the treatment of paraphilias is exhibitionism, which can be treated in an office setting. Men who feel an impulse to exhibit themselves are usually passive in their sexual pursuits, as well as in other areas of their lives. Despite the popular misconception of their dangerousness, exhibitionists are usually quite harmless, except in the psychological impact they may have on young women. The exhibitionistic experience provides an opportunity to exert power over a woman. The mere showing of the genitals and the subsequent surprise that the woman displays produce a feeling of power and sexual stimulation. The psychiatrist or psychologist tries to deal with the patient's lack of aggression with women. The patient is encouraged to be more aggressive in his general behavior and in his sexual pursuits. Often, these persons can change their behavior and have a more normal sexual life.

In contrast to the paraphilias, sexual dysfunctions often are treated in outpatient settings by psychiatrists and other psychotherapists. There are several ways to go about the treatment of sexual dysfunctions. The first is education. It is surprising how much misinformation is present in our society despite the marked increase in sexual activity in recent years. The psychiatrist first must be certain that the patient or couple is well informed about sexual matters. Through faulty information obtained in childhood or because of inhibitions about sex, many people do not know or understand how sex is supposed to happen. Every bookstore or library contains many volumes on the subject, but I am surprised how few of these books are read. It is hard to believe that the general public is still so inhibited about sex. It is more likely that people would rather pretend knowledge of the subject of sex than risk letting others know that they are uninformed on the subject.

In treating the sexual dysfunctions, the psychiatrist must first be certain that he or she is not dealing with a physical problem. If there is any doubt about a physical problem, a urologist or gynecologist should be consulted. Assuming that no such physical disorder exists, the preferred treatment is some form of psychotherapy. It need not be a long-term therapy such as psychoanalysis. Good success rates have been reported for short-term efforts.

In recent years, there has been progress in the treatment of sexual dysfunctions. Much credit for this progress goes to the pioneer work of William Masters and Virginia Johnson. In 1966, their first book, *Human Sexual Response,* described normal sexual behavior in better detail than had been done before. A subsequent book entitled *Human Sexual Inadequacy* contained information on the treatment of sexual dysfunctions. These books are considered classics in the field of normal and abnormal sexual behavior.

In their treatment protocol, Masters and Johnson treat the distressed couple daily over an intensive 2-week period. At first, any misinformation is corrected. Next, the couple is instructed to experience "sensate focusing" for several days. This technique is a nonsexual stimulation of body parts such as the arms, legs, and trunk. During this stage, the couple is told not to attempt intercourse or any direct sexual stimulation. After successfully exploring various body parts to find areas that are sensitive to touch, the couple is encouraged to touch the genitals and any other body part that is sensitive to sexual stimulation. The couple is told again not to attempt intercourse during this phase. Finally, the sexual act is attempted with the emphasis on enjoyment of the experience, not on success or failure of the act. The sexual act is viewed as a game that is to be enjoyed by both, with no winner or loser.

Psychiatrists have found Masters and Johnson's format difficult to reproduce in an office setting for a 2-week period. Some have adopted a longer and less intense version of the Masters and Johnson technique. In this variation, a couple is seen once or twice a week. The basic sexual education of the couple is first addressed. When the therapist is satisfied that the couple is sufficiently informed, the topic of sensate focusing is introduced. After the couple practices sensate focusing, stimulation of the sexual areas is suggested, followed by sexual play, which may conclude with some sexual experimentation. Intercourse may result, but again, the emphasis is on enjoying the moment and not on success or failure.

Case Example

Recently, I treated a married couple who was having sexual diffi-culties. Despite a relatively good marriage in many respects, Jane had never experienced an orgasm. This problem distressed her, and she felt inadequate. Her husband, Fred, felt that he was a poor lover because he was not able to bring his wife to orgasm. I treated the couple by the modified Masters and Johnson method. In less than 6 months, Jane had her first orgasm. She was quite pleased, although she did not have an orgasm every time that they had a sexual encounter. Neither Fred nor Jane felt that it was abso-lutely necessary that orgasm happen each time. The couple was satisfied with this level of improvement.

The Masters and Johnson technique assumes that the couple has minimal psychological problems. If the marriage is grossly troubled, the problems would have to be addressed first before this form of treatment could be applied.

Masturbation and Sexual Orientation Distress

Neither masturbation nor sexual orientation distress is considered a sexual disorder, and therefore they are not found in the official DSM-IV classification of sexual disturbances. However, each one is of such great concern to people that it deserves some discussion.

Masturbation

Masturbation is self-stimulation of the genitals. It begins in early childhood through experimentation with the pleasant sensations of touching the genitals. After puberty, masturbation often is accom-panied by ejaculation in males and orgasm in females. Masturbation has been blamed for mental illness, physical deformities, and loss of strength. Of course, none of these conditions is caused by masturba-tion. There is no evidence that masturbation causes any harmful physical consequences. But there still exists much guilt about masturbation, either based on religious beliefs that it is immoral or on neurotic guilt from childhood. The only abnormality associated with masturbation is when the act becomes compulsive and the person masturbates many times per day, in much the same way that a person might eat compulsively.

Results of Kinsey's survey published in the late 1940s revealed that virtually all men masturbate at some time in their lives, and about 75% of women admitted to masturbation. Masturbation often occurs when the individual is consumed with sexual tension and does not have a partner with whom to engage in sex. Although I have not seen written evidence for it, my guess is that masturbation often is used by paraphilic individuals as a way of avoiding sexual encounters; thus, masturbation is at times a means of preventing the paraphilia.

Sexual Orientation Distress

Some years ago, the American Psychiatric Association concluded that homosexuality was not an illness but a variation of normal sexuality, except if the state of homosexuality was distressing to the individual. There are many persons who are distressed with their homosexual urges, even if these feelings are not predominant over their heterosexual feelings.

Kinsey reported in 1948 that about 4% of adults were exclusively homosexual, and 13% were mainly homosexual for at least 3 years between ages 16 and 55 years. One in three men had at least one homosexual experience with orgasm after puberty. For women, the rates were about half those of men. Recent studies suggest that the rate of homosexuality is lower than Kinsey found, although popular magazines and newspapers give the impression that the incidence is far greater than Kinsey's statistics.

The cause of homosexuality has yet to be determined. Homosexuality is not commonly found in the animal kingdom when both sexes have access to each other. Why does it occur in humans? Hormone studies have yielded inconclusive results. It is known that in the prenatal days, the growing fetus requires sufficient male hormone for the male child to later prefer females as sexual objects. If the male hormone level is low, the adult male will prefer a male as a sex partner. Also, in twin studies, there is a higher incidence of homosexuality in one twin if the other is homosexual. In some families, there is a greater incidence of homosexuality among family members. These studies suggest a physical basis for homosexuality and possibly a genetic cause for these sexual preferences. Obviously, further research on homosexuality is necessary.

Sex and Society

In Western culture, sexual mores seem to change with each generation. In the last 50 years, there has been a revolution in sexual attitudes in this country. Has the change contributed to the well-being of our society or has it done harm? From the point of view of the freethinker and the sexual libertarian, it has been a favorable change, until AIDS appeared on the scene. Promiscuity of all sorts has not abated despite the rampant spread of this dreaded disease. Today, as I write about sex and society, a report appears in the newspaper that AIDS is now the leading cause of death among young adults, even exceeding accidents, and the epidemic shows no sign of abating. What are young people to do? Is safe sex the answer? Even if safe sex were the answer, is unbridled and unrestricted sex an answer to the satisfaction of our sexual needs?

Freud wrote that neuroses were caused by unresolved conflicts involving sex and aggression. Both sexual and aggressive impulses have been given much freer rein now than 50–100 years ago. Has this free rein produced a more content or healthy society? The answer is unclear. Of course, there is no going back to the last century, and many factors have contributed to the vast changes in our society.

Is it then the responsibility of philosophers, theologians, ethicists, mental health workers, and others to find answers to these questions? In my opinion, these groups can be of value in shaping the good of the culture. But it will take more than speeches and books to instill values among our society. The entire culture must bear responsibility for the problems that we face, including the media with their prurient and sensational interests and our educational system with its lack of concern for moral values. In addition, our governmental institutions must do more to stabilize the moral values of our society or give guidelines for moral direction.

What Can Families, Friends, and Caregivers Do?

Gender identity disorders are not easily treated unless discovered early. Families of those with gender identity disorders can help by taking their relatives to a therapist as soon as they recognize that the disorders exist.

Individuals who have paraphilias do not readily seek help from therapists unless it is court ordered. Family or friends can sometimes help by bringing these persons for help sooner. If the individuals accept assistance, they can sometimes be treated successfully.

There is considerably more help available for people with sexual dysfunctions. These individuals often resist seeking help, and that is the time when caregivers can be most helpful. The sexual partner of the patient may have to be involved in therapy as well. Understanding and patience are necessary for all concerned. Forcing someone to submit to treatment for a sexual disorder is of no use. Gentle persuasion may work. Sometimes it helps a patient to go to an internist or urologist for clarification that no physical problem exists before he or she will accept the help of a psychotherapist.

Sexual dysfunctions do not always demand a long period of therapy. The fact that symptoms have been present for a long time does not necessarily mean that help is not available.

CHAPTER 10

EATING DISORDERS

On occasion, I have wondered what would have happened to society if Freud had concentrated as much energy on the subject of food and eating as he did on sensuality, especially sexuality. My guess is that in child rearing, there is much more attention paid to eating and the problems that surround eating than to sexuality. How many arguments are there around the dinner table about Johnny not eating his food, not finishing what is on his plate? My estimate is that in most households with children younger than age 10 years, the food arguments in a family beat out the sex arguments by 1,000 to 1.

Just think what would have happened if the sexual revolution of the 1960s had been the "food revolution." What turn would it have taken? In my fantasy, I visualize the following: Everybody is now liberated and is eating anything they desire—without guilt. Gluttony is the preoccupation of the movies and TV, and sexuality is only a minor concern. No one is on a diet because eating is now a national sport. Society is becoming more and more creative with food fantasies. Some people are being jailed for forcing too much food on others. Numerous offenders are incarcerated for habitually looking in dining room windows while people are eating. Still others are criticized for exhibiting their food or eating habits.

This vision is a way of saying that if Freud had not raised the question about the impact of repressed sexuality on civilization, we probably would be looking at sexuality differently. Just how, I do not know. But in this country, there is a preoccupation with food, diets, and dining out, whether at fast-food restaurants or in expensive, well-appointed gourmet establishments. We all have heard the expression, You are what you eat. Certainly, nutrition is important, but you also are what you think and feel. It is equally urgent that you give attention to your thought processes and your emotional life.

Beginnings

The life of the fetus is entirely dependent upon the mother for sustenance. The umbilical cord supplies all of the nutrients that the fetus requires. If the mother is properly concerned about the quality of food she eats, the child will be born nutritionally healthy. At birth, the child depends on the mother for the basic foods for proper nutrition. The eating instinct does not have to be taught. If you touch an infant's cheek, it will turn its mouth in that direction (rooting reflex). The newborn is looking for the source of food. The touch suggests that food or its source, the nipple, is present in that direction. The sucking reflex need not be taught, as this too is an inborn reflex.

It is important that an infant be fed in a relaxed atmosphere by a mother who is not overly anxious or concerned about feeding. Problems surrounding food and the child's eating habits may begin early if the relationship between the mother and child is not sufficiently relaxed. Of course, there can be occasional exceptions when problems do not develop. American psychiatrist Harry Stack Sullivan maintained that the early relationship of the child to the mothering one in feeding, holding, and playing is vital to the child's future emotional health. He said that if a mother is tense, the child will pick up this tension. In effect, anxiety is contagious. A tense, anxious mother causes tension and anxiety in the child. This anxiety applies to all aspects of living. Anxiety in parents and other caregivers certainly does affect the child in all emotional relationships, including interactions at the family dinner table.

Changes in eating habits of children can be upsetting to parents. These alterations in eating are generally temporary, but the parental anxiety that it engenders can be harmful to children. The important issue is that the child is adequately fed over a period of time, not what he or she eats in a given day. If parents are obsessed with a child's eating habits, it can create a disturbed environment in the home. Forcing a child to eat certain foods or to finish all of the food on the plate is not advisable.

Overview of Eating Disorders

The most common eating problems encountered in our culture are obesity, anorexia (loss of at least 15% of ideal body weight), and bulimia (binge eating followed by purging). Oddly enough, obesity is not included in DSM-IV, even though it is more common than any other eating disorder. As explained in DSM-IV, obesity is not included "because it has not been established that it is consistently associated with a psychological or behavioral syndrome. However, when there is evidence that psychological factors are of importance in the etiology or course of a particular case of obesity, this can be indicated by noting the presence of Psychological Factors Affecting Medical Condition" (p. 539).

Obesity is not simply due to psychological factors; the emotional reasons for overeating in many people are undeniable. Most obese individuals are overweight because they enjoy eating. But there may be genetic and metabolic reasons for obesity as well.

Some women consciously or unconsciously prefer to be obese. They feel their obesity makes them less attractive to others, especially men, thus allowing them to avoid interpersonal relationships and conflicts about sexuality. Men often associate their obesity with power and strength; they feel more attractive that way.

As reviewed in the seventh edition of *Kaplan and Sadock's Synopsis of Psychiatry*, evidence from many studies shows that emotional problems are responsible for both anorexia and bulimia. Family dynamics are often involved and are discussed later in this chapter.

Generally, the eating habits and eating problems of children are affected by at least three factors: 1) parental attitudes toward food and discipline concerning eating, 2) peer pressure in childhood and adolescence about what and when to eat, and 3) changes in food, clothing (styles of dress, size and shape of clothing models), and health fads as advertised on TV.

Some studies on parental attitudes about nutrition indicate that overfeeding children can lead to obesity in later life. There are parents who are convinced of the idea that everything on the dinner plate must be eaten because that was the way they were taught. This attitude does not seem to be as prevalent now as in former generations, perhaps because it resulted from the worldwide depression of the 1930s and the famines reported at that time.

Peer pressure exerts a powerful effect on young people. Their eating habits are no exception. Fashions for young people have been greatly influenced by skinny models, such as Twiggy, for the last 25 years. But preoccupation with thinness is a recent phenomenon. Art history attests to the fact that well-endowed women were considered the ideal for many centuries. Today's youths regard being thin as beautiful. This viewpoint is particularly true among the upper and upper-middle classes. Many lower-class citizens and some ethnic groups do not share this view. It is my impression that with the emphasis on bodybuilding, which now also includes women, a more sensible attitude toward body shape and size will evolve.

Anorexia and bulimia are relatively new disorders. For example, when I was in medical school, I read about anorexia but never saw a single case until I was serving my internship. After that, it was some years before I had any patients in my private practice who had anorexia; it has now become epidemic. Bulimia probably has existed for centuries, but it was not described in the modern medical literature when I was in medical school. It is now asserted by some experts in the field that on college campuses 40% of the female students binge and purge at some time during their college years. Bulimia actually has become epidemic as well.

Early in my psychiatric practice, a young female patient told me that she vomited after meals to avoid gaining weight. To me, this was a strange new symptom because bulimia was not described as an illness until much later. She said that she ate everything on her plate at dinner, thus satisfying her parents. Then she went into the bathroom and vomited to satisfy herself, thus keeping her weight down. Since first hearing this story, I have encountered many other patients with the same problem.

It is interesting that bulimia and anorexia rarely occur among men, although the incidence of both disorders has increased somewhat among men in recent years. The image of the slender man is becoming more fashionable.

Anorexia and bulimia are rare not only among men, but also among the lower socioeconomic groups. In my work in an inner-city outpatient psychiatric clinic, I have been aware of the absence of bulimia and anorexia in our patient population, which is a low socioeconomic group. These eating disorders are seldom seen, even among the female population. Although this observation has been confirmed by studies among various socioeconomic groups, it is not known why this difference exists among low socioeconomic groups.

A common feature of anorexia and obesity is the phenomenon known as the distortion of body image. Individuals with a distortion of body image do not see themselves as others see them. If patients with anorexia look at themselves in the mirror or observe pictures of themselves in bathing suits, they see "fat" despite the fact that any other observer would see them as abnormally thin. Some patients describe feelings of revulsion at the thought of even the smallest amount of fatty tissue on their bodies. Among obese persons, there also is a distortion of body image, although it is not as striking as with anorexic persons. Obese individuals do not necessarily think of themselves as obese. A woman may consider herself to be pleasingly plump and a man well built or husky. Among individuals who have eating disorders, there is considerable denial about their body image. Denial is also obvious in discussions about food or diets with individuals who have eating disorders.

It may be hard for the average person to appreciate the degree to which body image can be distorted, but distortion is not so uncommon. For example, at one time, while looking at myself in the mirror, it appeared that I still had a full head of hair. But photographs of myself revealed my baldness and belied the image that was in the mirror. A colleague of mine reports the same experience.

A similar distortion applies to the process of aging. Some years ago, a 58-year-old patient told me that he could not imagine that he was that age. He said that he thought and felt about age 40. At the time, I found this statement hard to understand. But as I age, the truth of this observation has occurred to me as well. Few people feel that they are as old as their actual age. Our minds seem to have trouble keeping up with our chronological age. I have noticed the same thing happening with my athletic ability. Although old enough to know better, I sometimes feel unusually good about playing tennis or skiing—as though I were 30 years old. It's pleasant to have such fantasies about myself, but such flights of fancy can lead to excessive activity, strained muscles, and a sore back. Fortunately, the strains and soreness bring me back to reality, and I play sports in a way that is more in keeping with my age.

In patients who have eating disorders, their minds distort reality to a greater extent than those who have more common concerns, such as balding or aging. But it is surprising to me that there are not *more* eating disorders, given the fact that eating is such a delightful pleasure to most of us.

Classification of Eating Disorders

The major eating disorders of adults that are classified in DSM-IV include the following:

- Anorexia nervosa
- Bulimia nervosa

In addition to these major disorders, there is a category for eating disorder not otherwise specified. Although the most common eating disorder, obesity, is not classified in DSM-IV, there are many psychological components to this disorder. Despite its exclusion in DSM-IV, I discuss obesity in detail later in this chapter.

Anorexia Nervosa

Case Example

Some years ago, an internist asked me to consult with him about a 14-year-old girl who was in the hospital. He described his patient, Mary, as looking like a concentration camp victim. There was no physical disorder to account for her condition, only her failure to eat. She was of normal height for her age, but she weighed 60 pounds—far below the normal expected weight.

As I recall, this young patient was not very talkative or cooperative. It was difficult to get any important information from her about the onset of her anorexia. When I first spoke to her parents, they were not helpful either.

Although it was not yet a recognized treatment at the time, I knew that certain major tranquilizers and antidepressants made patients gain weight. I prescribed these medications and hoped that they would work. In the ensuing few days, she lost a few more pounds. After another week in the hospital, she and her family insisted that she return home. She had just begun to eat some food. My colleague and I felt that the discharge to home was premature, but we were not able to convince the family to have Mary remain in the hospital. I continued to see her in my office for treatment.

Mary was quiet and depressed. She was compulsive about her day and had a specific routine. She weighed herself daily and exercised strenuously to keep her weight down. Anything that interfered with her schedule made her angry. Mary spent time looking at herself in the mirror, looking for fat on her body. She had long given up on friends, as she was critical of them. Before her illness, she had had sufficient friends, but they did not seem to interest her now. She kept up with her work in school despite her illness. Her former interests in reading and sports were not now part of her day.

As time went on, I was able to get to know Mary a bit better. I involved her family in the therapy as well. Gradually, a picture of Mary and her family stress evolved. Mary had always been a perfectionist. She never seemed to be satisfied with her work or with what others thought about her. Mary's parents were puzzled about this and could not figure out a way to deal with her problems. As a young adolescent, she began to gain some weight, and one day a friend remarked that she was becoming fat. After hearing this remark, Mary went on a diet and promptly lost a few pounds, which seemed to end her concern about her weight. But a few years later, the obsession with her weight and the anorexia began.

From puberty on, Mary had problems dealing with the fact that she was developing physically. She felt ashamed of her breasts getting larger and was upset by family references to an aunt who was "hippy," meaning that she had excessive weight on her hips. Mary also was troubled by her attachment to her parents. One time when she was at a summer camp, she was homesick and wanted to come home. At other times, she resented her parents for telling her what to do and being too overprotective. Mary also had angry outbursts that seemed to be related to her frustration with her problems. In addition, her parents were quite restrictive of her behavior and overprotective of her.

Despite her view about weight, Mary gradually gained a few pounds. After about 6 months and with the continual use of medication, she reached 85 pounds. However, I never felt that Mary really understood the reasons for becoming anorexic. In the course of therapy, the communication with her parents improved, and she did appear to be more content. She began to socialize again, and her mood was more stable. Although I was not satisfied that I had thoroughly comprehended the emotional dynamics of her illness, I was pleased that she had made a clinical recovery. At one point at the beginning of her anorexia, her parents were afraid that she would actually die of the disorder. Their fears were not unfounded because a small percentage of anorexic patients do die. Fortunately, Mary recovered.

It is not uncommon for persons who have anorexia to carry their illness into adult life in a less severe form. Often, it is seen in combination with bulimia, especially as the person grows older. In general, it is easier to uncover the dynamics of the illness with older patients than with the very young.

There seems to be a relationship between anorexia and afflu-ence, since it is rare among the poor and in underdeveloped coun-tries. It is five times more common among females than males in some studies, and in others the ratio is even higher. Although, accord-ing to the definition in DSM-IV, anorexic patients must have lost 15% of normal minimal body weight, most lose much more than this amount. If a person loses too much weight, and there is no more fatty tissue to spare, the muscles begin to break down and the person ap-proaches death.

In addition to obsessions with eating and food rituals, some an-orexic patients consume diet pills and laxatives. They exercise exces-sively to lose even more weight. Furthermore, they may develop amenorrhea (failure to menstruate), excessive growth of hair on arms and legs, and heart problems. In females, the estrogen level is reduced, and thyroid disorders may occur. Among males, a low testosterone level is seen.

As mentioned previously, anorexic patients have a distortion in body image. When looking in the mirror, anorexic patients see fat all over their bodies. Furthermore, these individuals think in all-or-nothing terms. They see their family members and others as all good or all bad at any given time. This mode of thinking causes much emo-tional strife in the family and in other social situations. When hospi-talized, they are known to cause deep divisions among staff members by being able to polarize individuals into good and bad persons. In ad-dition to controlling their food intake, body weight, and physical ap-pearance, they also have a compelling need to control the people around them.

Anorexia can begin before puberty, although most cases start in adolescence. It can occur as a brief single episode, or it may become chronic and extend into adult life. Events such as moving to new loca-tions, going on a diet because of mild obesity, or tragedies may bring on anorexia. There is a high incidence of anorexia among ballet danc-ers, wrestlers, models, and jockeys, who diet to stay slim because of their occupations.

Anorexia is a serious disorder. Anorexic patients may become extremely depressed and sometimes suicidal. Some studies suggest that up to 18% of anorexic patients die; some commit suicide.

Causes of anorexia.   Anorexia is contrary to nature's demand to eat for pleasure and nutrition. How is it possible for a young person to become so consumed with looking thin that the obsession with eating and weight becomes dangerous to life?

Cultural aspects appear to play an important role in the occurrence of anorexia. Several generations ago, anorexia was known but was uncommon. The "thin" look is desirable at present, but styles change. One day it may not be fashionable to be slim. If this trend should occur, it is quite likely that anorexia will decline to levels that were present 50 years ago. In contrast, as people in the lower socioeconomic levels aspire to middle-class values in style and dress, there probably will be an increase in anorexia in this group.

One of the common problems among anorexic patients is dependence on parental figures. Although this struggle to gain independence begins early in childhood, it is particularly noticeable in adolescents as teenagers typically strive for independence while being dependent on their parents. This struggle is markedly exaggerated in anorexic patients. What appears to be stubborn behavior in anorexic patients is an unconscious attempt to deviate and separate from the wishes of the parents.

The fear of developing into a sexual being is a common problem for anorexic patients. They have difficulty coping with physical development, including breast size, changes in body contour, and menstruation. In addition, the new social roles that involve sexual orientation and interaction with peers, although challenging, often are fraught with fear. On an unconscious level, it is far safer to remain the little girl, who still looks the same as she did before puberty, than accept growing into an adult woman.

Authorities in the field of anorexia generally agree that the families of anorexic patients are dysfunctional in a number of ways, which may differ with each family. Among the problems are exaggerated closeness to one parent, an overemphasis on appearances, and parental difficulty with seeing the child grow up to become an adult sexual being. In addition, parents also have problems separating from their children and struggle with the dependence-independence issues.

Treatment of anorexia.   Among the important considerations in treating anorexia is nutrition. If nutrition is not appropriate, physical problems may ensue and death may occur. It is best to have a physician who is familiar with anorexia deal with weight and nutritional matters and a psychiatrist or other psychotherapist attend to the emotional factors. Having a physician and a therapist treat the patient is done because it is extremely difficult for a psychotherapist to treat the nutritional problems and the emotional difficulties at the same time. By separating the nutrition issues for the physician to handle, the therapist is left to confront the personal and family issues, which are large enough tasks.

If body weight dips too low and the patient reaches a physically dangerous point, hospitalization in a psychiatric unit of a general hospital is necessary to prevent complications. While the patient is in the hospital, the nurses will often divide their work into two parts. One group of nurses will attend to the nutritional aspects using behavior modification. Behavior modification involves giving rewards and punishments for behaviors surrounding food. Meanwhile, another group of nurses and other therapists can deal with the personal and family problems of the patient.

Both in a hospital and an office setting, medications often are helpful in treating anorexic patients. In extreme cases, medications may even be lifesaving. For reasons that are not well understood, antidepressant medications stimulate appetite and thereby help anorexic patients to eat. Also, most patients who have anorexia are clinically depressed, and these medications may help the depression as well. Major tranquilizers such as Thorazine (chlorpromazine), Navane (thiothixene), and Haldol (haloperidol) also increase appetite and are useful for treating anorexic patients.

Individual therapy is used to increase self-esteem and ferret out personal problems that may be present. Family therapy involving one, two, or all family members enables the therapist to understand and help with troubled family interactions. All of this therapy usually is not done in a few sessions. It requires months and years to treat anorexia adequately if it has become a moderate or severe problem. Borderline or mild anorexia can be treated in office settings by psychotherapists if patients are brought in for treatment early enough.

For those anorexic patients who are learning about the illness, there are support groups located throughout the country that exist to educate and give emotional assistance. These low-cost groups are helpful to those who are open to learning about anorexia once they have even partially accepted it as an illness. I encourage patients with anorexia to attend these groups on a regular basis.

Bulimia

Patients with bulimia eat copious amounts of food, far beyond what would be required by ordinary hunger or nutritional needs. This excessive eating is followed by either fasting or purging. Purging is done by inducing vomiting or diarrhea in order to eliminate the ingested food. Although this behavior probably has existed for centuries, it was not described in the medical literature until the 1950s. Persons with bulimia may be normal weight, anorexic, or obese.

Bulimia is now known to be common, especially among college students. If a young person vomits infrequently after gorging, it may not result in a serious condition. However, if persistent purging occurs, it can result in physical complications that are important. Frequent vomiting can cause ulcers of the esophagus and an electrolyte disturbance in the blood. It also results in the destruction of the tooth enamel. It is not unusual for a dentist to be the first one to suspect bulimia in a young person, since it is an illness that is often kept secret.

Some bulimic patients binge and purge many times a day; others may do so weekly or less often. It is known that bulimic patients also may drink excessively, ingest a variety of drugs, steal, and become depressed and even suicidal. The emotional and behavioral patterns of bulimic patients are viewed by therapists as not unlike the drinking and drug behaviors of young people. In its mild form, bulimia is assumed to be "normal" behavior in this age group.

Research on this disorder shows that bulimic patients who are of normal weight often are hungry even after eating a reasonable amount of food. Their experience of hunger is different from the norm. For some unexplained reason, they also use calories in a more efficient manner than others.

Causes of bulimia.   Why are there an excessive craving for food and an excessive need to purge? Experts on the subject of bulimia have suggested that the disorder has to do with unsatisfied sexual needs or fears of sexual encounters. The need to stay slim and conform to the current cultural standard has been stressed. It has impressed me that in some cases bulimia represents, among other things, the desire to please parents by eating and please the self by purging. Another speculation is that bulimic patients try symbolically to expel the unwanted parts of the self. Perhaps this is true in some cases, but each individual must be helped to discover his or her own emotional dynamics rather than be fit into a particular psychological theory.

Two cases of bulimia.   Bulimia is well known to many people now. As a result, more patients now are seen earlier in the illness than in the past.

Case Example 1

Judy, a 19-year-old college student, admitted to occasional binges and purging on a weekly basis. For about 6 months, the symptoms had become more frequent when she was going through emotional problems with a male friend. Judy was of normal weight, but she had a tendency to gain weight if she let herself go. She consciously controlled her weight by vomiting. However, vomiting was uncomfortable and distressing to her. She wanted to stop the bulimic symptoms and look into any other possible motives that she might have for the recent onset of bulimia.

In all other aspects of her life, Judy appeared to be doing well. She was an excellent student, had formed goals for herself, and had an active social life. She also reported an intact and well-functioning family. I later confirmed these facts by talking with her parents.

Despite her success, Judy was somewhat shy and had a low self-esteem. After some months of weekly psychotherapy sessions, she felt better about herself and was able to control her food intake in a more realistic and practical manner. The bulimic symptoms were not easy to give up, but her control over them was eventually strengthened. Would she ever relapse? Possibly, but she was no longer in any danger of bulimia taking charge of her life.

Case Example 2

Joan was a 15-year-old who had been bingeing and purging for 4 years. Joan's symptoms were severe, and she had developed ulcers in her esophagus. Much of her tooth enamel had been worn away, requiring considerable dental care. Besides the bulimia, Joan had been drinking and using drugs for at least 3 years. In many areas of her life, she was out of control. It also was apparent that her parents had little control of her behavior. Because of the severity of the illness, Joan had to be hospitalized in a setting that specialized in bulimia and could deal with her other emotional and behavioral problems. Joan had to remain there for about 6 weeks to make some sense of her disorganized life. When she returned home, she had to face up to her addictive behavior by attending an Alcoholics Anonymous (AA) meeting regularly. In addition, she joined a group for people with anorexia and bulimia. In my office, I conducted family therapy to deal with her personal and family difficulties. It was not an easy task. It took years of concerted effort to turn around Joan's life, but she did make it. Her low self-esteem and her unmet emotional needs and goals for her life were addressed. In addition, her family members eventually were able to see how their involvement also contributed to Joan's problems.

Treatment of bulimia.   Some studies show that the antidepressant Prozac (fluoxetine) appears to be quite useful in the treatment of bulimia.

Obesity

If we are at least 20% above our ideal body weight, then we are officially considered to be obese, according to authorities on the subject. By this standard, many of us are obese.

But what causes obesity? We all know people who eat copious amounts of food and never gain weight. In contrast, there are individuals who eat relatively little, exercise regularly, and still gain weight. What causes this phenomenon? It is not simply a matter of calories consumed; rather, obesity is due to a complex combination of metabolic, hereditary, and psychological factors. Just how all these elements bring about obesity is not well understood, but we know more now than before because of the research on obesity that is being done.

Obesity is more common in women than in men. In this country, it is found more frequently among first-generation ethnic groups. Statistically, obesity is especially high among Hungarians, Italians, Czechoslovakians, and the British. Among religious groups, statistics show that obesity is highest among Jews and appears to be lower among Catholics and lowest among Protestants. The reasons for these variations are not known.

Metabolic factors.   There is good evidence that metabolic factors play a part in obesity. Low thyroid function (hypothyroidism) is associated with obesity. Certain pituitary and adrenal disorders also can induce obesity. More research is needed in this area.

Hereditary factors.   Obesity is known to be hereditary. In 40% of cases, if one parent is obese, the adolescent children are obese. If there is obesity in both parents, the children will be obese in 80% of cases. In contrast to these observations, if children live with obese adoptive parents, there is no higher rate of obesity in these children. This finding supports the idea that heredity plays an important part in the development of obesity. A friend of mine told me that he has never left the dinner table without the feeling that he could still eat more. As you might expect, he is obese. One theory on obesity is that obese people react to a greater degree to the sight and smell of food. In contrast, persons who are not obese do not have this tendency and are more apt to eat when they are hungry.

Psychological factors.   In some families, there is an excessive concern with eating. Food may be equated with love, and overfeeding may be thought of as evidence of love. In some societies, an abundance of food may be viewed as evidence of prosperity and success. In America, there is a high value placed on slimness, because of the current styles, especially in the middle and upper classes.

In an attempt to explain obesity, Freud and his followers theorized that obesity was based on exaggerated dependency needs. The presumption is that these needs were not met sufficiently early in life. Obese individuals seem to put a high premium on satisfying their oral needs. Yet, despite this observation, recent research shows that obese people do not have significantly more psychological problems than the average person. On the other hand, few obese individuals feel good about being "fat" and may have a low self-concept. Some suffer from a distortion of body image. These concerns appear to be the result of obesity and are not involved with the origins of the illness.

Physiological theories on obesity.   There are two main theories that have been recognized by researchers. One is the fat cell theory, which states that there are two times in a child's development when fat cells are deposited in the body—at age 2 years and again from ages 10 to 14 years. Once these fat cells are present, they do not go away, although they may increase or decrease in size. Persons who have accumulated a large number of these fat cells in childhood are apt to be obese adults. This theory has led to the idea that overfeeding children is conducive to obesity in later life.

The other theory on obesity is the set point theory. Animal experiments reveal that if overfed or starved, animals usually return to their original weight—their set point. Although animals have a set point in their weight, and a set point has been observed in some humans, it is not always true for variations of human weight. When humans diet and lose weight, it appears hard to maintain this lower weight. Most people eventually return to their former higher weight. By contrast, when humans become obese, it is difficult for many to go back to their set point.

Other body functions also account for variations in body weight. In the lower part of the brain, called the brain stem, there is an appetite center that controls the feeling of hunger. It is influenced by a variety of factors by means of neurotransmitters, the chemicals that carry messages to other parts of the brain. Additional factors affecting hunger include the state of the gastrointestinal tract with its enzymes and the presence of illnesses such as cancer.

Obesity and effects on health.   In both men and women, there are illnesses that are associated with obesity. These include gallstones, gouty arthritis, and osteoarthritis. Heart disease, high blood pressure, and increased serum cholesterol and triglycerides also occur with obesity. In addition, hyperinsulinism (with low blood sugar), which often occurs with obesity, can be a forerunner of diabetes. In men, obesity is associated with impotence and a decreased interest in sex. In women, polycystic kidneys, abnormal hair growth, and menstrual irregularities may be seen with obesity.

Treatment of obesity.   As most of us know, dieting is not easy, and it is hard to maintain a desirable weight. Is it willpower, determination, or some other mental trick that is needed? Most people who diet eventually return to their former weight. Only about 5% are able to remain at the level that was obtained through dieting.

In recent years, calorie intake has not been emphasized as it had been previously; rather, dieters have been advised to reduce fat intake. Reducing fat intake has been shown to be more helpful than has been calorie counting. Thus, lean meats, white meats, and fish are recommended. Pasta and bread are low in fat but do have substantial calories. These foods are now being suggested along with plenty of fresh fruits and vegetables.

There are several medicines available to help reduce appetite. They may be helpful when first beginning diet programs, but they do not help much in consistent appetite control. Two that have been commonly prescribed are Pondimin (fenfluramine) and Tenuate (diethylpropion).

There are other methods that are useful in helping individuals lose weight. Behavior modification and hypnotism, by trained therapists, are sometimes used. But such help should be considered only in addition to dieting, not as a substitute for it. Weight Watchers groups have had a good record in supporting the efforts of those on diets. Weight Watchers uses a form of behavior modification and group support. Overeaters Anonymous also is successful for dieters; this group uses the 12-step program of AA. Some studies indicate that psychoanalytically oriented psychotherapy also has helped patients with obesity, particularly those who have low self-esteem or poor body image.

Exercise has been stressed much more in recent years for controlling body weight because it decreases appetite and increases body metabolism. Exercise appears to be less helpful for losing weight than for preventing further weight gain. But for exercise to be really effective, a person should work out at least three times per week for 30 minutes. Exercise alone without dieting will do little to help a person lose a significant amount of weight.

Surgical intervention is sometimes recommended for severe obesity that does not respond to other treatment methods. This type of surgery is risky and involves bypass operations or gastric stapling. These procedures permit less food to be ingested and absorbed. This surgery is a specialty in itself and should be done only by physicians with considerable experience.

Lifestyle changes.   Losing weight is not the hardest of tasks, but maintaining the desired weight is extremely difficult. What is necessary for the more or less permanent control of obesity? It requires more than willpower and determination. It involves a firm commitment and a genuine change in lifestyle.

Case Example

I have a friend named Frank. He happens to be a professional person. As far as I can understand the issue of obesity, I think he has the best control of the problem that I have seen.

Some years ago when I first met Frank, he was very obese, not just a little overweight. I knew him as a respected colleague. I saw him perhaps once a month at our staff meetings. One day, it occurred to me that Frank looked quite different. He had lost a considerable amount of weight. I hesitated to ask him about this change until sometime later, but my curiosity had been piqued. I asked Frank to tell me how he was able to lose his excess weight.

It was an interesting story. Frank had lost more than 100 pounds, and in the last several years, he has been able to maintain his desired weight. Frank told me that he eats three meals a day without snacking. He eats far less at each meal than he has ever done before. He eats food that is nutritious and low in fat. Frank has adopted a new philosophy on the subject of eating. He eats enough to live and feel well, eating because it is necessary but not because it represents to him a time for oral satisfaction and gluttony. He made eating a small but necessary part of his life while giving priority to other things, such as the enjoyment of music, art, and reading.

Frank revealed to me that his family placed a high premium on eating. It was one of the more important times in the day for the family. His mother had forced food on him and clearly gave him the idea that eating was central to life. Frank tried to reverse this basic message learned in childhood; he now eats to live rather than lives to eat—and he is succeeding.

I know of no better way for anyone to be as thoroughly in control of eating. It takes a totally new way of viewing food and satisfying the appetite for food. A lifestyle change is necessary, but that requires a change in attitude in dealing with one of life's great pleasures.

What Can Families, Friends, and Caregivers Do?

The family is especially important in dealing with anorexia and bulimia. Attitudes toward eating, as well as attention to emotional problems in the family, are essential to consider although not easy to change. The biggest problem for the patient as well as the family is denial of the disorder, that is, denial that the family and the patient have together created the problem, not denial of its existence. It is not important to argue whether the primary problem belongs to the patient or the family. Both are intimately involved. It is virtually impossible for patient or family to solve these eating problems unassisted. It is important for them to be motivated and seek outside help from a psychiatrist or other mental health specialist who has had experience in treating eating disorders.

Family and friends of the obese patient can be extremely helpful. When a person begins dieting, it is useful to avoid having a supply of high-calorie and high-fat foods around the house. Encouragement and support by family and friends are of prime importance. Dieting for the obese individual is a serious business and should not be taken lightly. Through dieting, a great source of pleasure is being altered.

Other sources of pleasure, interests, and new experiences should replace eating, although these may be difficult for many individuals to find.

Persons on a diet need all the help they can get from their family and friends. It is difficult for obese individuals to deprive themselves of their favorite pastime. It is hard to diet in isolation without considerable support.

As with anorexic and bulimic patients, obese patients usually have some psychological problems. It may be necessary for the whole family to seek help in understanding how they contribute to the problem of obesity. For example, some mothers are obsessed with their children eating enough. They tend to overfeed their children and feel fulfilled only if the children are overweight. Attention to proper nutrition may be part of the therapy with the family.

CHAPTER 11

THE EMOTIONAL EFFECTS OF LOSS

I am certain that you have noticed a sense of fulfillment and satisfaction when you have helped someone in distress. It feels great when your help is appreciated, but when your assistance is not accepted, you feel let down. You usually experience this feeling as a minor loss. I feel this way when a patient comes to see me and does not continue beyond a few visits, offering a reason that does not seem convincing to me. Although this example represents a minor loss, if it occurred frequently, I would have to ask myself if I were working in the right field.

Some losses have a great impact on the individual, whereas others have relatively little. If a friend does not share my good fortune with some enthusiasm, I feel a sense of loss. In contrast, when I am in deep emotional pain because of the illness or death of a loved one and my friend does not acknowledge my pain, I feel anger or hurt that my loss is not appreciated by him or her.

For example, one day, as I entered the hospital to visit my 17-year-old son who was suffering from leukemia, I met a friend who is a physician. He asked me how I was doing. I replied that I had come to the hospital to visit my son. He immediately asked if I was going to a medical meeting that was being held that day. He knew about my son's illness but was completely unable to relate to my pain. Although I resented it at the time, I later granted the possibility that my friend could not bear the thought of such an illness striking one of his children; he simply could not talk about it.

I was surprised indeed that many of my friends could not bring up the subject of my son's illness. Were they trying to protect me from pain, or were they avoiding pain themselves? I am certain that this response varies with each person, but I experienced my friends' lack of communication as an emotional loss and a failure by them to give me support. Oddly enough, if I offered information on my son's condition, some people usually were able to talk about it. His illness then seemed like a safe topic. I am certain that this attitude is familiar to anyone who has been in a similar situation, such as having a close relative who has a serious psychiatric illness.

I have known losses—the death of both parents, two older brothers, and a sister. But the loss of elderly parents or older siblings does not feel the same as the loss of a child. It has been more than 20 years since our 17-year-old son died from leukemia. After a 2-year illness, during which he fought bravely and continued with school and sports, he finally succumbed to this dreaded disease. The loss at first was great, as I had expected, but the recurrent pain felt over the years was more than I had anticipated. Even now, certain emotional situations that occur in conversation or in a play or movie can revive the pain, if only briefly. How do you accept the unfulfilled life, the dashing of hopes and aspirations, of your child? Some individuals lose their whole families in fires, accidents, or other calamities. These tragedies represent the ultimate losses to me. Perhaps to some individuals there are other losses that are more devastating.

Loss is felt differently by everyone. It depends on the nature of the loss and how it impacts a person's life. For example, someone who has $20 million and loses a million may not feel a great loss. However, if a person is extremely insecure about money and measures his or her life's worth only in terms of net worth, he or she may be extremely upset by the loss of that $1 million.

Not everyone is grossly disturbed by the death of a spouse. Many a difficult and distressing marriage has been immediately resolved by the death of one of the partners. I do not mean this facetiously. It is difficult to feel deep mourning for a husband's death if he does not occupy a strong emotional place in the mind of the surviving wife.

Another example is the loss of a job. Some people react to this loss as though it were the end of life. Others feel quite casual about it and feel optimistic about getting a new job. Some even welcome the idea of new employment or even changing their careers.

All physicians are aware that their patients handle illness in different ways. Some time ago, a physician told me about two of his patients who were diagnosed at the same time with the identical disease, a form of cancer. The first man intellectualized the whole process and became an expert on the illness by reading everything he could find on the disease and its treatment. He never appeared upset or distressed about the illness or his impending death. When the physician told the second man about his cancer, the man went into a depression that lasted throughout his illness until his death.

How Do We Defend Against Loss?

Physicians, nurses, and other caregivers have long been aware of the sense of loss that is experienced with illness and death. They also have been aware of the depression, anger, and disbelief that people often express when dealing with illness and death. Freud was one of the first to contribute to this subject in a paper he wrote in the early 1900s. It contained helpful ideas about the difference between the process of mourning losses and the clinical state of depression or melancholia, thus the title "Mourning and Melancholia." Freud contended that in both mourning and depression, people usually repressed considerable anger that was not consciously recognized. He felt that in treating persons distressed by either of these conditions, it was necessary to help them become aware of their anger in order to facilitate recovery. This discovery by Freud was significant, and the idea of uncovering repressed anger is still used by psychotherapists in treating depression or prolonged grief reactions. But Freud did not elaborate on the other defenses that occur with these emotional states.

Only in recent years have these emotional reactions to impending death been so clearly understood. In an excellent book, *On Death and Dying*, Dr. Elisabeth Kubler-Ross spelled out the various stages of the process associated with serious illness and death. She detailed the defenses people use to cope with dying and the prospect of death. Gradually, the insights from this book have been integrated into the medical community, and health care workers have come to accept and use this knowledge in their work with dying patients. One of the outgrowths of her work has been the hospice movement.

It should be noted that the defenses people use in reacting to death and dying are similar to those used when people experience any significant loss. Other significant losses and corresponding reactions are discussed in detail later in this chapter.

Kubler-Ross described five stages that most individuals go through in dealing with death and dying. These stages do not follow in an exact sequence. Some people go through the stages quickly, some may skip one stage or another, and others may remain in one stage for a long time and pass through other stages quickly. The reactions to death and dying affect people in different ways, but the following five stages usually can be recognized:

1. *Denial.*   If you have ever faced the threat of a serious illness or the prospect of death, you probably know about denial. It is a state of disbelief: "How could this be happening to me? I just can't believe it. I know this happens to others, but I never dreamed that it would happen to me."

   Although denial is a common first response to bad news, it is remarkably absent in some people. The ultimate realists among us say that they want to face whatever is wrong and need to know everything about their illness or future. They seem better able to cope with the reality of death and dying. But most people use denial when first confronted with the possibility of death. Denial is an unconscious defense mechanism that occurs automatically and not by choice. It need not be present all the time. A person may deny the significance of his or her situation one day and be realistic about it the next day. The intensity of denial may be mild or may reach unrealistic proportions and actually become delusional. For most people, denial serves a good purpose. It serves to relieve the individual of the stress of the immediate impact of bad news. Denial can occur not only in the person who may die but also in the family or close friends of the affected person.

Our minds have a wonderful way of repressing bad news as well. I am certain that you have had the experience of being obsessed with the painful reality of a serious calamity that you recently learned about. But even on your worst days, you found yourself momentarily forgetting about the traumatic situation. Your mind repressed the thoughts. Repression is necessary so that you can cope with and attend to the affairs of life while you go through a difficult period. Denial, however, is not forgetting about the pain but actually not believing that it exists. It is a temporary state of disbelief.

Does everyone want to know about impending death? I have known friends who were never told of the seriousness of their illnesses. In one case, neither the physician nor the family notified the person of his cancer. He had a major operation and survived for about a year. At no time did he ask about his illness or his future, despite his obvious loss of weight and continual poor health. Some people do not want to know what is going to happen. Others must know.

Denial is a normal healthy reaction to the stress of impending death. Caregivers can see through denial, but it would be a mistake to interfere with it until the person is ready to stop the denial. There is an exception. If an obvious successful treatment is available for the illness and the person refuses to accept it because of his or her denial, the caregivers and the physician should try to break through the denial to avail the person of the treatment.

2. *Anger.*   Anger may occur after a period of denial, or it may happen soon after the threat of death. Anger may have several sources. Some people are angry because they have a long list of things that they had planned to do. The illness that they have

obviously will interfere with plans such as achieving certain job-related goals, financial plans, or traveling. Others are angry because they do not accept the fact of illness or the threat of death as happening to them. The questions Why me? and What did I do to deserve this? keep recurring. Without denying the facts of the situation, they are angry that this fate has come upon them.

The anger that occurs at times of illness and impending death may be directed against the very people who are caring for the ill individuals. The anger may be excessive or even irrational. It may be related to a feeling of helplessness during severe illness or thoughts of death.

Some persons have little anger; others have an excessive amount. Some pass through this stage easily, whereas others never seem to be free of anger. It depends on the basic personality of the person who is ill. Caregivers should be aware of the necessity of anger in the dying person and should try to be patient with its expression. Today's anger may become tomorrow's depression or resignation. Time is required for this change.

3. *Depression.*   Life has a way of getting us down. It may be as simple a problem as fatigue that can bring on depression. When there is a loss, depression eventually strikes the individual to one degree or another. When a person cannot deny possible or actual loss or gets angry at the way fate, or God, or circumstances have brought about loss, then depression is likely to occur. As Freud pointed out, when anger is turned inward on the self, the mood is lowered, energy levels are depleted, and the affected person slows down, sometimes to a virtual stop. Sleep is difficult and normal appetite disappears. Even immunity to various diseases is lowered when depression is present.

The degree of depression associated with loss may be mild to severe; it can even make some individuals suicidal. When people must handle serious illness, suicidal ideas are not uncommon. If individuals lose considerable wealth or their homes, they may feel so despondent that they think ending their lives is the best way out of the dilemma. If a caregiver notices that a person is talking even in vague terms about harming himself or herself in any way, the idea of suicide should be considered. When suicidal ideas are noted, an experienced mental health specialist should be consulted.

Frequently, depression associated with loss is limited to a short time. But I have seen it last for years, for example, when a person loses a loved one or loses a job that he or she is not able to replace with a new position.

As a patient, relative, or friend goes through the stages of anger and depression, it is important for the caregiver to be a good listener. There is no advantage to giving a lot of advice to someone when he or she is so distressed. It is essential to listen carefully and to try to feel empathy for the angry or depressed person. However, it serves no useful purpose to listen for hours late into the night to an angry or depressed individual. The caregiver should end the listening after a sufficient time, an hour or two at most.

In addition to being good listeners, caregivers should act with a degree of firmness. When a person is depressed, caregivers might suggest, "Move your muscles. The worst thing you can do is lie in bed all day." Or if the person is talking endlessly about something, it is helpful firmly to end the conversation and suggest another activity.

When caregivers deal with someone who is depressed, the work can become extremely frustrating. Caregivers can become annoyed, irritable, or angry too. If such feelings are a reaction to the continual demands of the depressed individual, firmness is again the route to take. There is a limit to the tolerance of caregivers. When this limit is reached, the depressed person should be made aware of it. When caregivers express annoyance or frustration, it often has a positive effect on the depressed person. Somehow sensing dependence on the caretaker, the depressed individual becomes more cooperative, if only for a short time.

4. *Bargaining.*   After individuals know that they are dying, they may deny the situation or be angry and depressed. But at some

point, they may try to bargain with fate or God and essentially say to themselves, God, if you save me from this illness, I will do the following for you. These individuals then promise to give money to worthy causes, volunteer their help, be better people, or whatever comes to mind. Bargaining is a mental attempt to right the situation through a transaction, a quid pro quo with God. When bargaining occurs, people usually become much calmer, as though they have more control over the problem.

5. *Resolution.* The resolution stage may occur early in the process of dying, but more often it comes at a later time. When the individual feels that death is inevitable, he or she may have some peace of mind about it—a resignation to the facts of dying. When this resignation occurs, it may be interrupted for short periods by anger or depression. Resolution may be accompanied by the person's arranging his or her affairs properly for family members and others. The person then may decide to die with some degree of dignity and make his or her last wishes known. Meanwhile, occasional episodes of anger and depression may intervene. In fact, all stages may be seen in any given day, only to change on another day.

The five stages described do not run sequentially but may occur at any time, except for denial, which usually does come first, and resolution, which comes last.

Stages of Grief in the Family

Although a person dying goes through the five stages outlined by Kubler-Ross, these stages also can be observed among the family and close friends of the dying individual. The persons most intimately involved with the dying one are the most likely to be affected by strong emotional reactions. These emotions can be similar to the five stages through which the dying person progresses. I distinctly remember passing through all the stages more than once while our son was dying and after his death.

I have observed patients who became stuck in one stage or another. Some, after learning about the impending death of a loved one, deny the possibility of death for a long time. Others get caught in the anger stage, whereas others are overwhelmed with depression.

Case Example

One of my patients, Joe, became extremely depressed after losing his wife. Before her death, I had seen the couple for marriage counseling. Marital disputes occurred during the therapy sessions as well as at home. They were critical of each other, and at times the arguments were quite bitter. At other times, they appeared to have good feelings toward each other. Then one day Joe's wife, Mary, suddenly died from a stroke. At first, Joe went through a short period of disbelief. He did not become angry in any way but became depressed and remained down. He failed to go through the normal grief reactions that are now commonly recognized.

When I talked with Joe in our therapy sessions, he only had the grandest compliments for his wife. She was hailed as the best person who ever lived on earth; she deserved sainthood. When asked about their marital relationship, Joe could only focus on the wonderful times they had together. He could not relate to the anger and hostility that were present during their marriage. He completely denied these emotions. At one point, he became so distressed that I had to consider hospitalization. Joe expressed suicidal thoughts but did not appear to be overtly suicidal. I continued to treat him at my office.

In addition to his denial about the anger and hostility present in his marriage, Joe also could not get in touch with his anger toward Mary for suddenly leaving him in such pain. This reaction is part of normal grieving in most people, but with Joe it was markedly exaggerated. Failing to recognize his anger kept him in a continual state of depression. I had to point out to him that I had heard about the bitter fights that he and Mary had at home and witnessed them in my office. Gradually, he began to realize that he did have negative feelings toward Mary. In time, he saw Mary in a more realistic light: a loving person who had many fine qualities but who also possessed human frailties. With psychotherapy and medication, Joe improved. His suicidal ideas disappeared, and he started to function more appropriately. Within several months, he had recovered from the depression and had good as well as sad memories of his departed wife.

In some elderly persons who lose their spouse, the anger never is expressed, and these unfortunate people remain depressed for years. For some, separation through death is difficult; for others, it appears to be more easily handled. I have found it hard to predict how a patient or friend will react to the loss of a close friend or relative. The individual variations in behavior are truly remarkable.

Other Losses

Does everybody go through the five stages of grief each time that they experience a loss? No. If the loss is minor, some individuals may become irritated and mildly depressed and may walk away from the situation feeling no worse for wear. When mild losses occur, some people handle them with healthy defense mechanisms. For example, if a person loses a job with which he or she was not happy, the person may rationalize the loss, saying to himself or herself that he or she really did not want the job anyway and that other jobs are more interesting, probably pay more, and have greater prestige. Or the person may become angry about a job loss, blame his or her boss and others who were involved, and justify his or her actions regarding work. After the anger has been sufficiently expressed, he or she may accept the situation, particularly if a new and more satisfactory job is obtained.

We also experience loss when we lose power, self-esteem, wealth, or anything that is of value to us. Sometimes, rather insignificant losses can have a profound effect on people. It depends on how much emotional investment they have in that which is valued. I have seen people mourn for months over the death of a pet or the loss of an inexpensive piece of jewelry that had some sentimental value. Sometimes, people become depressed over the failure to get a raise at their job or when they are not acknowledged for relatively small accomplishments at work. These losses may be followed by all or some of the five stages of grief. Bargaining, however, may not occur with less significant losses and is mostly seen in losses associated with death and dying.

The following examples are typical of losses that are commonly seen by psychiatrists and other mental health workers.

Work

Some jobs become obsolete, which certainly happened to the blacksmith as the automobile became more prominent. But it seems to happen even more swiftly now than in the past. For example, not many years ago, most secretaries were expected to be proficient at using the office typewriter. Then the computer arrived on the scene. With this new invention and its magical mysteries came a degree of fear and apprehension on the part of its users. Most secretaries made the adjustment and learned to deal with the computer. Even the computer manufacturers recognized the emotional reactions to the new invention and created user-friendly software. But for those who could not make the adjustment to the new era, there was a sense of loss if not the actual loss of a job. Others became computer operators and programmers. However, the field developed so fast that yesterday's knowledge was soon outdated. If workers did not keep up their skills or learn the new programs and techniques, they fell behind and became rapidly obsolete. They lost their positions at work or had to go to a job where less was required of them. I have known persons who have suffered such losses. Anger and depression were common reactions.

Early retirement is another situation that can be experienced as a severe loss.

Case Example

Fred was 56 years old when he came to see me because he could not deal with feeling so angry and depressed that his company had retired him prematurely. He had planned to work until age 65 and then retire with sufficient pension to move to a retirement community in North Carolina. He and his wife were looking forward to this time. The children were grown and doing well on their own. As long as Fred had his full pension, financially he could live comfortably in his retirement years. But now he had to stop working 9 years before he had expected, thereby reducing his pension benefits.

Fred's first reaction to the news of early retirement was disbelief. How could his old reliable company do this to him after all these years? The company was known to be considerate of its employees. But times had changed, and the large companies were cutting back—downsizing. At first, Fred became angry at his boss, who was not in a position to do anything about the downsizing because the decision did not originate from him. It was company policy that had been determined at a higher level. Fred realized that his boss was not the problem, and he could not vent his anger at any one person—it was that damn company! He soon became depressed. All his plans were suddenly destroyed. What would he do now? "Getting a job at my age for the income I was receiving isn't easy, Doc," Fred said. I empathized with his plight, but the reality was that Fred had to make a major adjustment in his plans for the future. Getting another job would be difficult.

As the weeks passed by, Fred became increasingly agitated along with his depression. His despair reached the point that he longed to escape. He thought about suicide but said he did not have "the guts" to do it. I treated him in my office and gave him one of the newer antidepressants, Prozac (fluoxetine). After about a month of taking the medication, ventilating his anger, and talking about alternatives to his situation, Fred began to feel somewhat better. It took about 6 months before Fred felt well enough to see his problem as a challenge rather than the end of the world. Fortunately, Fred had 6 months' severance pay to tide him over to the time when he could consider alternative jobs. The job he finally got did not have the prestige or power of his former position, but he eventually accepted the change and made a satisfactory adjustment. He planned to work a couple of years beyond age 65 and then retire.

As so often happens in life, the best-laid plans do not always work out on our timetable. Illness, accidents, and many other unforeseen events frequently intercede and force us to alter our dreams.

One way to think about loss is to see it as a separation problem. For example, loss can occur with death, divorce, job, or money. Separations occur at many stages of life. Loss of security is common in the child when he or she misses Mother. Later on, some children experience great anxiety if they are left in nursery school or kindergarten. As a consultant to public schools, I frequently saw children of all ages who were afraid to go to school. These children with school phobia were not as fearful of school as they were of leaving the security of home. Even later, when going off to camp or college, children often become ill and have to return home. Some remain dependent and never want to leave the security of home. They do not want to leave the familiar and the comfortable. (For more information on issues of separation, see Chapter 2 in this volume.)

Divorce

Many couples who are divorced have literally mourned the loss of the relationship for such a long time that by the time they are divorced, there is no genuine loss to be handled. But some couples fail to go through all the stages involved with loss and continue to be depressed and angry. Persons in these relationships may even attempt to remarry each other. I have seldom seen these remarriages work out successfully. Generally, if a couple has not been able to resolve some reasonable fulfillment of their mutual needs in marriage, they rarely are able to do it with a second try with the same person. As a rule, too much emotional damage has been done for the two to feel kind toward each other long enough to repair the marriage.

Even when individuals divorce and have no intention of remarrying each other, there may be a sense of loss. Memories of the children as youngsters or when the couple was happily engaged in pleasant activities may bring on feelings of loss and questions of why the divorce had to occur. Although divorce represents the failure of a relationship, there may have been many wonderful times in the early part of the marriage. In nostalgic moments, a deep sense of loss can be brought to the surface.

Power

The ascent to power is a heady experience. Most people who attain power in their work-related activities do so gradually as they obtain promotions over the years. In the world of politics, it can occur dramatically. I can attest to this from a personal experience. After one unsuccessful attempt running for the United States House of Representatives against an incumbent, my wife, Marge, succeeded on the second try. On the very first day in office, she arrived early before any of the office staff. The telephone was ringing, and she answered it. A constituent from the district was calling about a family member who was lost in a Central American country. After hearing about the problem, she contacted the State Department and talked with a number of officials. She proceeded through the hierarchy to the top levels. Toward evening she was on the phone with the secretary of state. After a detailed conversation, the secretary of state told the new congresswoman that she should call the family involved and inform them about their discussion of the problem and tell them what had been learned thus far. She politely suggested to him that the call would be more meaningful if it came from him; he agreed to do the calling.

When Marge told me this story, I was quite impressed. Just days before, she was wife/mother/community activist, and on that day she was attempting to assist a family with an international issue and suggesting to the secretary of state how he could best perform his job. This sudden elevation to power astounded me.

During the last 12 years since this event took place, I have seen many powerful political figures fall from high positions. We all remember, some years ago, Watergate and the downfall of Richard Nixon. I have seen many congressmen and senators lose their positions through electoral defeat or through irresponsible behavior.

Defeat is hard to take, although some individuals seem able to resolve it better than others. Many rationalize defeat as bad luck or blame others for their misfortune. Some become depressed or have symptoms related to their emotional state.

Whether the loss is one of prestige, influence, or position, it represents a loss of power. Once a person has experienced power, it often is hard to give up, even when it is done voluntarily.

But not everyone is enamored with power. Many people avoid it. They fear the responsibility of power and prefer the lesser role of assisting those in charge. They are followers rather than leaders. Some function much better in such secondary roles.

Possessions

I have known people who are attached to their homes. Leaving home even briefly is difficult for them. I have seen a few persons become depressed by leaving one home and moving to another. A home often provides considerable security to people, especially to older persons. But some can move about freely from one place to another without much distress. They do not seem to need the security that a home provides. Perhaps it suits them better to move on and make new acquaintances; the physical home is of little importance to them. In the 2 years I spent in the military service, I met marines and navy personnel who had made the military their career. They were forced to move to a new base about every 2–3 years and it did not seem to bother them. They had friends on other bases, and they looked forward to seeing them. The new home to which they were moving was just another necessary but unimportant part of being a military person.

Some people find security in hoarding possessions, whether money, antiques, artwork, property, or any other tangible objects. When such things are lost or stolen, it has a profound effect on these persons.

Independence

Another loss that affects some more than others occurs when people enter a hospital for a period longer than a few days. I have seen some people respond badly to the fact that they are forced to become dependent on the nurses and physicians for everything. The dependence makes some feel helpless, particularly aggressive, impatient, independent type A personalities, who pride themselves on not needing anyone. I also have known patients who seem to thrive on the attention that they receive while in the hospital. One person's loss appears to be another's gain.

Function

Loss of function may be experienced in many ways. Accidents or illness may cause physical defects that limit physical functions. Emotional or mental illnesses may prevent people from functioning in a variety of ways. Some traumas are so overwhelming that the individual has a total inability to function at all for a short time. This inability to function is certainly true for those who have any major mental illness such as a psychosis. In depression, for example, the loss of functioning may be partial or complete depending on the severity of the depression.

Accidents cause physical and emotional pain and disabilities. The inability to perform well at work or at what had been enjoyable hobbies or sports may be felt as a terrible loss. With accidents, there is an additional factor involving financial compensation for the accident. Long legal battles and frequent physicians' examinations sometimes impede a person's progress toward health. While the victim of the accident deals with the loss of function, family members may resent the loss of services that the individual had performed as part of the family. Thus, the accident victim may have to deal with both his or her loss of function and the anger generated in the family.

Several years ago I suffered a loss of function for several months. For the first time in my life, I was hospitalized for cardiac surgery. A defective aortic valve had calcified over the years and had to be replaced. The surgery went well, the care was excellent, and my family was very supportive. But I was not able to work at all for about 2 months.

Before the surgery, I had read that in the early days of cardiac surgery about 30% of patients experienced depression postoperatively. As cardiac teams became more alert to this fact, they were able to reduce this to 5%. My experience was good; I had no depression, even though I was out of commission for a few months. However, I had started a program of regular exercise after leaving the hospital. This program suited me fine as I had exercised regularly before the surgery. After about 3 months, I noticed that I had reached a plateau. The level was not anywhere close to what I was used to before the surgery. When I tried to ski at a familiar location, I became aware of my severe limitations in terms of strength and endurance. Breathing was difficult and slopes that I used to handle with ease were now major challenges. These limitations were not exactly a boost to my self-esteem, nor did they create any optimism about the future. I soon noticed a mild depression. It was not enough to interfere with my work, but it was definitely there. Fortunately, this mood change did not last long, as I gradually became stronger. Since that time, most of my physical abilities have returned.

How Do People Deal With Loss?

We all handle loss in different ways. It depends on what significance the loss has to us. Some people have trouble handling even minor losses. Others seem to survive major losses with little difficulty. In addition, one loss may be tolerable, or even two, but some unfortunate persons must undergo one severe loss after another until they are crushed by the sheer amount of loss that they have to bear.

One of the first steps a person can take is to share the loss with someone else—a friend or a family member. If the loss is mild, it is helpful to ventilate the concerns to another person. Sharing feelings with someone may be all that is necessary.

Without even being aware of it, our ego usually begins the work of dealing with loss in the absence of our specific direction. We begin to deny the loss, rationalize the problem, or repress the significance of the loss. Or we may blame others for our fate and become angry at them for causing our loss. These defenses may be enough to deal with the problem. If not, it may be necessary to go through the five stages associated with loss.

When I talk with individuals who have sustained significant losses, I like to ask the following questions: What can you do about the situation that you are not doing? What changes in your life could make the loss more tolerable? What other advantages would occur if the changes were made? Is there any positive side to the loss? What do the feelings about the loss tell us about you? It is not uncommon that after an important loss, some people are better off than they were before the loss. For example, I remember talking with a man who had lost his job. He was terribly distressed and angry about it. Within a few months, he had obtained a new job, which turned out to be a much more satisfactory job than the previous one, even though he was not earning quite as much money.

Ultimately, we must all adapt ourselves to our losses as they come to us throughout life. Failure to adapt may result in chronic depression or anger. For example, recently, I talked with a patient who cannot seem to free herself from the past. She is not able to deal with the malevolent treatment that she received from her parents when she was young. It haunts her even now at age 55; she cannot put the past behind her and live her life with any degree of contentment.

For those who are grieving severe loss or are having difficulty reacting to moderate losses, a psychotherapist may be helpful. If the loss involves religious concerns, the appropriate clergyperson should be consulted as well. In our society, the value of the clergy is often overlooked and ignored. Many people are embarrassed to ask for help from the clergy, as though they are admitting a deep fault or weakness.

For those who are grieving the loss of a loved one and are not able to go on with their lives, a grief recovery group may be helpful. These groups are now available in most major communities as self-help groups. I also recommend a book entitled *The Grief Recovery Handbook* by John W. James and Frank Cherry. In this book, the authors describe the various losses that people can endure throughout life and suggest that grieving persons list all the losses that have occurred to them. They make the point that people are taught to acquire objects, possessions, and friends in childhood but are not taught how do deal with loss. Thinking about past losses and recalling the ways in which these losses were handled may help some people in recovering from a current loss.

The authors also mention myths about grieving that are common to our culture, including the following:

- You must replace what was lost with something or somebody.
- It is best to grieve alone.
- Time will cure you.
- It is best to bury feelings.
- Because of past losses, it does not pay to trust.

The authors strongly suggest that persons not grieve alone but share their grief with others who also are grieving. My own view is that for most people, sharing grief with others is extremely helpful, but for a few people, it is difficult to share what they feel with someone else. Some seem to have to go it alone. However, I think an attempt should be made to share the feelings associated with grief with other grievers or with close friends or confidants.

James and Cherry describe one kind of griever as showing "admirable restraint and poise" and call these reactions "Academy Award" recoveries. Individuals who have such reactions do not usually do well in the succeeding months after their loss. Often, the grieving is prolonged for many years. Some of these individuals become clinically depressed and need psychiatric care. Antidepressants, hospitalization, and even electroconvulsive therapy (ECT) may be required.

A legitimate question can be raised about treatment for someone who has experienced a loss. How can a medication or any other therapy do anything to cure a severe loss such as the loss of a loved one? The answer is that when serious depression occurs, there are biochemical changes in the brain. The neurotransmitters that carry nerve impulses from one nerve to another are lowered, thus causing the whole depressive syndrome. Even the immune system is weakened. When antidepressants or ECT is used, the neurotransmitters return to normal and the person feels improved. At this point, the patient is better able to cope with life. Although the patient is still aware of the loss, he or she may see the loss from a different viewpoint.

What Can Families, Friends, and Caregivers Do?

All of us have sustained certain losses, some more than others. Does this experience make us all experts in dealing with loss? No, but there are ways to help and be supportive. As mentioned earlier in this chapter, some losses are more profound than others, depending on the person involved. There are losses that are hard for me to understand. For example, the loss of a pet affects some people deeply.

Not being an ardent pet lover, it is hard for me to feel the grief of those who have lost a pet, unless I think of it symbolically as equivalent to losing a child, in which case I can relate to the mourning.

There are several suggestions that I feel are valid for helping the person who has suffered a severe loss.

Listen to the griever. He or she has the need to tell you in detail how the loss occurred. There is nothing that is more helpful to the person in mourning than to have a sympathetic listener. He or she has to retell the story over and over again. It may be repetitious, but interrupting the retelling can be distressing to the griever. Time is important. Provide enough time to do the listening, and listen with interest and compassion, without immediately telling the story of your own loss. The griever does not need to hear that you had a similar loss because he or she is in no emotional state to sympathize with you at that point.

Don't worry about what to say. Err on the side of saying too little. Long speeches and pep talks are not needed or desirable. Just give support and offer help. A bag of groceries or a meal gives physical support to your offer of help.

If you find that your support is of little help and the griever is remaining in a state of mourning far beyond the usual time, seek outside help from a mental health specialist. Some caregivers have a need to prove themselves helpful to anyone in any situation. Psychotherapists are aware of this tendency within themselves and have to be alert to it. We call this phenomenon rescue fantasies. The rescue fantasy consists of unconscious desires to be the rescuer, the only person who can help in the crisis—the mental health equivalent of the Lone Ranger.

Most people do not have answers about what a person should do when he or she experiences a loss. Being a matchmaker for the widow, widower, or divorced person may not be appropriate. If someone loses a job, quick suggestions about a new job may not be timed right. If you are going to make definite suggestions, don't be in a hurry to do so. The person who has experienced loss needs your support more than your advice.

When talking with a friend or family member about loss, it is important to keep in mind the possibility of suicide. Although no one can predict with complete accuracy whether a depressed person will commit suicide, the potential must be considered and help obtained if necessary.

In addition, grieving persons should be helped to make decisions about doing things that they formerly found pleasant. But progress usually has to be made in small steps. If improvement suddenly occurs, it will be because the grieving persons are able to do something for themselves, not because of the help that they obtained from those around them. There is a limit to what caregiving can do to help those who have suffered loss.

CHAPTER 12

PERSONALITY DISORDERS

We all have unique personalities, and none of us are exactly alike in the way in which we behave or express ourselves. We see a variety of personalities within our own families or at our places of work. Certainly, I see many different personality types in my office.

Case Example

Several years ago, I was asked to consult with a high school student nicknamed Bud. His parents gave me the following information on the telephone: Bud had always been a pleasant boy. He never gave his parents any major problems, except for his schoolwork. He scored in the 90th percentile in math and verbal tests, but he was failing in his academic work. Obviously, this scenario frustrated his parents greatly, and they wanted me to examine him to see what could be done about his motivation for school.

When I interviewed Bud, he seemed pleasant and agreeable. He readily admitted his failure to succeed at school, but he also said that he liked school. He enjoyed the many friends he had there. He happily participated in sports, although he was not a star athlete. Bud was polite and ingratiating; no teacher ever had a harsh word to say about him. However, in each succeeding grade, the teachers said that Bud had the ability but he had difficulty applying himself to his work. They were equally frustrated in trying to help him succeed.

His parents and friends noted that at the beginning of each semester he vowed to do better, and during the first month or two, it appeared that he was applying himself. The first-quarter grades showed a B average. His parents and friends commented on the change in Bud and his renewed attention to his schoolwork. Then the slide began. Before the semester was finished, Bud would manage to get his grades down to the D-average level. However, he never allowed himself to go so low that the grade represented an absolute failure, and each year the same thing happened.

With this pattern of behavior occurring regularly, Bud was sent to be evaluated by the school's child study team. After careful testing for learning disabilities, the team concluded that he had the ability to perform well in school but that he had emotional or personality problems preventing him from doing so. The child study team referred him to me for treatment.

Although always agreeable to therapy and any comments I made about his behavior or personality, Bud initially remained unmoved by the therapy or any attempts by his parents to alter his attention to school.

Psychiatrists refer to the pattern of behavior Bud exhibited as passive-aggressive behavior. Every psychiatrist is familiar with this pattern, although it is not classified as a disorder in DSM-IV. Bud, for example, was agreeable and conforming in his demeanor on the surface, but by being passive, he resisted his parents and teachers. A passive-resistant mode prevented him from progressing appropriately. Emotionally, Bud consciously conformed to the wishes of those around him, but unconsciously, he expressed his anger at being made to do things. With his massive resistance to any request, including simple chores around the house or work at school, Bud managed to get back at his parents and teachers because of their demands. Meanwhile, Bud was only dimly aware of the fact that by behaving in this manner, he was jeopardizing his own future. He had the potential to do well, enter a good college, and choose a future career to his liking.

Another patient with a similar passive-aggressive personality pattern once told me that he felt that he was being sucked into a giant funnel in having to make choices about schoolwork, college, and his future. He tried to resist this pressure in every way possible and delayed making his decisions for many years.

With Bud, my task in therapy was to develop a relationship with him without making demands on him, with the exception that he show up for his appointments. After 2 years in treatment, Bud was finally able to understand that he was doing himself a disservice. As he put it, "I'm cutting my own throat by not doing what is best for my future." He began to realize that if he did well in school, it would be primarily for his welfare and only secondarily would it please his parents. Furthermore, he gradually understood that his behavior was an unproductive way to express the normal anger that every adolescent feels toward his or her parents and school, as well as society in general. He gradually was able to express feelings more directly with friends and family in a way that was effective. Whereas formerly his anger was acted out in his resistance toward school, he now was able to express anger appropriately when he felt the need to do so.

Did all of Bud's passive-aggressive traits change? No. However, he was able to alter his behavior enough to succeed in school, but he continued to do battle with the residual traits of procrastination and postponing responsibility.

What Are Personality Disorders?

According to the seventh edition of the *American Psychiatric Glossary*, personality disorders are "enduring patterns of perceiving, relating to, and thinking about the environment and oneself that begin by early adulthood and are exhibited in a wide range of important social and personal contexts. These patterns are inflexible and maladaptive, causing either significant functional impairment or subjective distress" (p. 153). Persons with personality disorders are known to bother others greatly by their irritating ways. In contrast, persons with neurotic disorders are troubled and stressed by their own condition; they usually do not affect others adversely. To have a personality disorder, by definition, the person involved must be at least age 18 years. In a younger individual, any specific behaviors are referred to as personality *traits* rather than personality *disorders*.

It is important to distinguish between personality disorders and neuroses. The former are lifelong patterns of behavior that represent the unique personality of the individual. Neuroses, by contrast, are disturbances that develop sometime during adolescence or adult life, appear rather suddenly, and may last a short time or become chronic. Furthermore, neuroses are characterized by an emotional conflict and result in symptoms such as anxiety, depression, amnesia, phobias, and psychosomatic symptoms. For example, individuals with obsessive-compulsive personality disorder show unusual concern with cleanliness, money, possessions, time, and completing tasks in a particular way—their way. It is difficult for obsessive-compulsive persons to leave tasks undone (e.g., leaving dishes in the sink, cutting only half of the lawn). These individuals keep their records in perfect order, are always on time or early for appointments, and know exactly how much money they have in the bank. They tend to be exacting about everything.

People who have neuroses are struck by symptoms that are frightening. The symptoms may appear as sudden anxiety or an overwhelming depression that incapacitates the individuals. Symptoms are usually brought on by a conflict between the wishes of the individuals (id impulses) and their conscience (superegos) and the wishes of others. (For further discussion of the neuroses, see Chapter 7 in this volume.)

Formation of the Personality

The debate about the importance of heredity versus environment has gone on for centuries. Beginning in the first part of the 20th century, through the influence of Freud's writings, much more emphasis was placed on the environment and early parental influences, almost to the exclusion of hereditary factors. More recently, the importance of heredity has been confirmed by researchers, although parenting is still relevant.

Heredity appears to be a factor in children's temperaments, for example. Important research findings by Thomas and Chess were published in 1977 in their book entitled *Temperament and Development*. They began with healthy newborn infants in hospital settings. Each child was evaluated daily at first and then less often as time went on. The 141 children in the study were followed for 20 years, and the findings were interesting. At least three kinds of temperament were identified, all of which continued to be evident throughout the years into adult life. The researchers referred to the child's temperament as "behavioral style." About 65% of the children showed one of three behavioral styles. The remaining 35% had mixed behavioral styles.

One group of children was quiet, content to sleep a lot, and easily satisfied. These children, even as infants, cried only when hungry or when they had some physical need. This group, consisting of 40% of the children, was the largest of the three groups, and a child in this group was referred to as the *quiet child.*

The second group was the smallest, consisting of 10% of the children. These children were loud, cried frequently, and slept little. They were usually heard above all the others. This group also remained much the same behaviorally into adult life. A child in this group was called the *difficult child.*

The third group consisted of 15% of the children. Youngsters in this group did not throw themselves into activities with others until they were certain that they would be accepted. They were cautious about entering new situations, whether a bath, a new school, or any other new experience. Once they were involved in a group or activity, they became good participants. A child in this group was called the *slow to warm up child.*

As these children were monitored over the 20 years, they tended to continue to show their same behavioral styles, with few exceptions. Severe psychological problems or stressors caused a temporary change in behavior in some, but these children usually reverted back to their behavioral type after the stressors or problems were no longer present.

What other factors influenced the behavior of the children? Thomas and Chess mention "goodness of fit" of the temperament of the child in relation to his or her parents. For example, an active, boisterous child who grows up with quiet, less active parents who prefer to read, watch TV, or enjoy quiet activities at home do not form a good fit. These parents would have difficulty coping with such a child's behavior. They would find it hard to understand the child's nature and deal with all the hyperactivity. Conversely, active parents who are highly sociable may find it hard to deal with a quiet child who prefers to sit and read books and seems to have little need for friends.

Why was this study important? It gave some scientific evidence that there were inborn temperaments that tended to stay the same throughout life. This observation was in marked contrast to the psychological theories implying that parenting was the sole determinant in how a child develops and behaves. Thomas and Chess explain, "As mental health professionals we became increasingly concerned at the dominating professional ideology of the time, in which the causation of all child psychopathology, from simple behavior problems to juvenile delinquency to schizophrenia itself, was laid at the door of the mother" (p. 5). In the past, most inferences about children were made by studying adults and analyzing what may have happened to the children through experiences with parents and the environment. These so-called retrospective studies are subject to much bias and faulty conclusions by the observers, depending on their theories about human behavior. Furthermore, the memories of adults about their childhood are known to be slanted by feelings and are subject to a variety of interpretations, thus the many schools of psychoanalysis. In contrast, the research of Thomas and Chess is prospective and draws conclusions based on observations made over time. This type of research tends to be more scientific in its conclusions.

Temperament is a behavioral style, the energy or driving force behind individuals. The various personality traits, such as overreaction to stimuli (e.g., temper tantrums) or minor obsessive-compulsive behaviors (e.g., lining up dolls or cars), can be seen early in the behavior of toddlers. In studies of identical twins reared apart, an amazing number of personality traits were found to be similar. Even their interests, jobs, and hobbies had a sameness about them. This finding suggests that personality traits are at least partially inherited. Although it has not been proven that all traits are inherited, it seems evident that basic temperament, inherited traits, parenting, and environment all go together to make up the final personality.

Classification of Personality Disorders

DSM-IV lists 11 personality disorders. You may recognize some of them among your friends or family members. I describe the various personality disorders listed within three groups called clusters. Those who have any one of the personality disorders do not necessarily need to have all of the characteristics listed in order to be diagnosed as having a particular personality disorder.

Cluster A: Odd and Eccentric

Paranoid personality disorder.   People with paranoid personality disorder are suspicious and distrustful and doubt everything. They find it hard to believe anything people tell them. They are negative and usually expect the worst from others. When a person treats them well, they become suspicious of that person's motives. Because of these traits, they do not form friendships easily. Furthermore, they become angry easily, and they tend to alienate others; poor interpersonal relationships follow.

Schizoid personality disorder.   Those who have schizoid personality disorder daydream often and are quite lonely. They are withdrawn and may appear to be emotionally cold, rarely showing changes in mood or enthusiasm for things.

Schizotypal personality disorder.   Individuals with schizotypal personality disorder may appear eccentric and strange to others. These individuals may be preoccupied with psychic phenomena, may claim to be clairvoyant, and may speak of the physical presence of persons long dead. There are strong beliefs in magical thinking and superstitions and little regard for logical thought. Although people with this type of personality disorder may be interesting, they develop few good friends.

Cluster B: Dramatic, Labile, and Erratic

Antisocial personality disorder.   People who have antisocial personality disorder engage in behaviors that are disapproved of by society. They may commit crimes such as stealing and murder, or they may be con artists and extort money from innocent people. They often abuse drugs and alcohol and have few close friends because they tend to use people for selfish purposes. They are irresponsible and impulsive. Those with antisocial personality disorder have a poorly developed conscience, and as a result, they do not learn well from previous experiences. Furthermore, these individuals seem to have little or no remorse about their antisocial acts.

Persons with this personality disorder usually have a history of truancy and petty thievery when young. They experiment with sex and drugs prematurely. Poor performance in school is the rule. They are known to be cruel to animals and sometimes to other children. They have difficulty being truthful and honest with others.

Borderline personality disorder.   People who have borderline personality disorder are generally impulsive, and they tend to think in black-and-white terms. They react extremely emotionally to people in their environment. They may adore someone one day and hate him or her the next, which occurs to a greater degree than is normal. These individuals have problems with sexual orientation and may be confused about their sexual role. Occasionally, they may have "minipsychotic" periods that require brief hospitalization. They often idealize others and are disappointed when these individuals show signs of being human. Their tendency toward erratic behavior leads them into drug and alcohol abuse and excessive sexual acting out. Those with borderline personality disorder have difficulty maintaining close interpersonal relationships.

Histrionic personality disorder.   Those with histrionic personality disorder speak and act in extraordinary ways. Females usually have this disorder, but occasionally, males do as well. Every emotional experience that happens to them appears to be of equal importance. Things are always *the best* or *the worst*. These individuals are concerned with appearances. They seek praise and cherish constant approval. They are seductive in their behavior and usually are not consciously aware of this quality. There is a strong need for quick gratification of any felt need. Persons with this disorder, by virtue of their vivaciousness, may be quickly attractive to others, but generally, they often have troubled relationships with other people.

Narcissistic personality disorder.   Individuals with narcissistic personality disorder do everything for number one. They are not concerned with others but are out to gratify their own needs. They are grandiose in their wishes and demands and feel entitled to things that others would not think about. They expect to be praised and noticed for doing little, and they fantasize that they are more important than what others would assess. They use people for their benefit and lack feelings for those around them. With all of these negative traits, they still may wonder why they are not liked or even adored.

Cluster C: Anxious and Fearful

Avoidant personality disorder.   People with avoidant personality disorder are phobic about social situations. Shyness, fear of criticism, and embarrassment when in the public arena are typical. Fear of showing any emotion in front of others and fear of being ridiculed are characteristic. As a result, these individuals have few friends.

Dependent personality disorder.   Those with dependent personality disorder fear being alone. They do not like to take responsibility for things that others assume without difficulty. They fear criticism and are wary of being wrong about anything. Individuals who have this disorder rely heavily on the goodwill of others and do not dare to alienate those on whom they depend.

Obsessive-compulsive personality disorder.   Individuals who have obsessive-compulsive personality disorder are perfectionists in the tasks they perform and in their interpersonal relationships; therefore, they may expect perfection of others. They are overly concerned with time, money (miserliness), and cleanliness. As a result, they may be excessively concerned about how they look and how well they perform. These individuals are usually too conscientious and may be overly scrupulous. People with this personality disorder intellectualize emotional situations and are not good at expressing feelings.

Personality disorder not otherwise specified.   Personality disorder not otherwise specified is the term used when individuals have personality traits that are abnormal but do not clearly fit into any of the other classifications of personality disorders.

The Psychiatrist and Patients With Personality Disorders

How do psychiatrists fare in handling patients who have difficult personality disorders? Not as well as we would like. First of all, people who have these disorders usually are not bothered by their personality disturbances; rather, their exaggerated personality traits bother those around them. Unlike neurotic individuals, who have symptoms such as anxiety or depression, people with personality disorders do not readily seek help from a psychotherapist because they are not often in emotional pain, but they certainly can be a pain to those around them. When such individuals do ask for help, it is because they are in situations where someone can no longer tolerate their behavior. For example, if a supervisor threatens to fire an employee with a disagreeable personality, that individual may seek help because of fear of losing his or her job. Therefore, one kind of crisis or another may lead these persons to treatment. Although they may want help to deal with the crisis, they generally do not request that their personality be altered in any way. It is then up to the psychotherapist to decide whether modifications in behavior are possible or whether personality change should be a therapeutic goal.

What Can Families, Friends, and Caregivers Do?

Sometimes it is more harmful than helpful to label persons as having a specific type of personality. It may cause observers, including professionals, to identify the type and thus pigeonhole individuals, not allowing for other more positive personality traits to emerge or be seen. However, having more knowledge of someone's personality allows the possibility of understanding another individual better.

If you have friends or relatives who seem to have any one of the personality disorders, it may be useful to keep in mind that the various traits that make up personality are long-standing patterns of behavior and are not likely to change. It is easier and more productive to work with or around the particular personality traits rather than hope those traits will be dramatically altered.

One of the best examples of someone with a personality disorder can be seen on the TV program *The Odd Couple*. The character Felix Unger has many of the qualities seen in obsessive-compulsive personality disorder (e.g., cleanliness, perfectionism, and never being satisfied with a job not done in accordance with his standards). At the same time, he has histrionic traits (e.g., always wanting to be the center of attention and overreacting to people and events). This combination of obsessive-compulsive and histrionic traits makes him an interesting character. Oscar Madison, the carefree, sloppy gambler and cigar smoker, is in many ways the opposite of Felix. One of the themes of the show is the constant attempt by Felix to change Oscar, to make him over into Felix's own image. "Oh, Oscar, Oscar, Oscar!" laments Felix, as if to say, "Why can't you be a neat, clean, concerned, conscientious person like me?" The failed attempts to do so are what makes the show interesting and enduring.

A similar scene is repeated many times in real families in which one member is constantly trying to change the other through one form of pressure or another. A mother trying to make a Felix out of her sloppy son and an intellectual father trying to make a good student out of a passive-aggressive daughter are examples of this interaction.

Should there be no attempts to change a family member or friend? No, but expecting major changes in personality is quite different from requiring certain modifications in behaviors. The following three case examples illustrate how behavior modifications would work in therapy or when caregivers must deal with certain personality disorders. The three case examples are patients whom I have known. I had to consider the various personalities involved in order to work out a therapeutic solution. In the three general examples that follow the case examples, I describe how caregivers can work with individuals who have other personality disorders.

Case Example 1

When I was involved in marital counseling, I encountered one couple in which the husband, an exacting, scrupulous person, was extremely busy at his job, which prevented him from doing the basic monthly task of paying the family bills by check. He assigned this job to his wife. She had all the earmarks of histrionic personality disorder. She expressed herself in exaggerated ways, made ordinary events seem like major calamities, and, of course, failed to ever balance the family checkbook. Her husband became furious at her inability to keep financial matters in order and insisted that she "do things right." Despite all his complaining to her and his many suggestions, she was not able to complete her task. Monthly fights about finances were common in this family.

It may be obvious that the wrong person was in charge of the checkbook; however, the couple did not readily see this as the problem. The husband kept insisting that he was too busy to balance the checkbook and that his wife had more time. But having more time was not the essential element in getting the job done. It took some convincing, but the couple eventually made a simple change. The husband discovered that in only a half hour every 2 weeks, he could take care of the finances and do it well. His efforts prevented many needless arguments. The couple had to learn that a histrionic person should not be expected to do accounting, just as it would have been a mistake to expect the busy executive husband with his obsessive-compulsive traits to plan the interior decorating in the home. Everyone has strengths and weaknesses. Family jobs should be assigned to those capable of completing them well.

Case Example 2

Recently, I encountered a young woman, Bethany, who had married three times. Her previous two husbands were different individuals, but both had many unfortunate character and behavioral problems. The other two husbands had one thing in common with her present husband: they all had aggressive personalities. Bethany recognized this trait in all of them and said that she always had been attracted to aggressive men. After several sessions, she began talking about her father and his charming nature. As she told me more about him, it became obvious that he may have had many wonderful qualities, but he also was extremely aggressive, a quality about which Bethany was only dimly aware. When this fact finally dawned on her, she became upset and cried profusely. She now realized that although she was attracted to aggressive men, once she married and had to cope with them, she had a poor track record. However, there was one difference. Her current husband was a good provider, and he was generally good with the children. With the exception of his overbearing ways, which sometimes frightened them, he did show appropriate affection toward them. Considering all of these positive qualities, she was not about to leave him and seek a divorce. What was she to do? She lived with someone who had an aggressive personality, but how could she manage always feeling as if she were the object of his anger and aggression? This problem is why Bethany sought consultation.

I suggested several possibilities. One was including her husband in the therapy, either in joint sessions with us or in individual sessions with me. I also suggested that Bethany talk with her husband about her problem of feeling horrible about his aggressive ways, with the hope that he might moderate his aggression toward her to some degree. She chose the latter path. I continued to see her in weekly psychotherapy sessions. In the course of 6 months, she learned to counter her husband's aggression in small ways. She also developed a thicker skin, a way of reacting to his aggression that was not devastating. She learned not to let some of his typical aggressive remarks affect her, which she had not been able to do before. Meanwhile, her husband reduced his aggressive impulses enough to make the marriage more tolerable. Together the couple worked out the problem. About a year later, Bethany called. We had a review session, and she reported that things were going okay, not perfect by any means, but okay. I was satisfied that my patient had learned to cope better with her husband's aggressive personality and satisfied with her husband's simultaneous modifications in behavior.

All caregivers encounter patients with borderline personality disorder at one time or another. Individuals with this disorder are among the most difficult to help. Caregivers in all fields are confounded and stumped by the incredible maneuvers of patients with borderline personality disorder.

Case Example 3

I was called to consult with 30-year-old Jean in a local hospital. When I first met her, Jean was pleasant enough, but it did not take long before I learned about her anger toward certain members of the staff. She thought some of them were not worthy to be called nurses, whereas others were the very reincarnation of Florence Nightingale. No caregiver on the unit occupied neutral ground. Jean idolized her physician, who was an internist. He could do no wrong. Similarly, she spoke in superlatives about some of her friends, all of whom were relatively new, while condemning all of her old friends. Her parents did not fare well in her opinion either. She was not easily satisfied with anyone for long. I learned from Jean and her physician that she was impetuous, was confused about her sexuality, and had a tendency to become depressed often, although never for a long period. On occasions when she was despondent, she cut her wrists lightly with a razor, being careful never to do any serious damage. Several times, Jean had been admitted to a hospital because of feeling suicidal, which was the reason for her present admission.

Jean was not an easy person to help. I consulted with her physician about her background and her basic personality. He was aware of her problem and wanted to know what to do with Jean in the hospital. He wondered whether the hospital could actually help her. I explained to her physician that Jean had a most difficult personality and that only the greatest amount of patience would help her in the long run. I told him that although Jean idolized him now, he should expect to be denounced as a failure one day and should not take it too seriously. I told the nursing staff that Jean is the kind of person who tends to polarize any staff, whether in a hospital or at her place of employment. I suggested that they accept the fact that some of the nurses would be viewed by Jean as incompetent, whereas others would be adored. If they understood that this was Jean's nature, they hopefully would be less offended by her remarks.

I agreed to see Jean for psychotherapy when she left the hospital. I knew therapy was going to be difficult. She had many periods of emotional turmoil. I tried to be the person on whom she could rely, even if she insulted me or ignored my suggestions. After several years in a stormy marital relationship, Jean steered her way through the difficult marriage and found a more suitable spouse who was able to roll with her emotional waves. As time went on, her difficult personality traits became more moderate and she was able to live a more productive life. Years later, she wrote to me about her success with her family and a small business that she had started.

Although personality traits are enduring, they tend to moderate with age, as was the case with Jean. Understanding the nature of her personality and what to expect from her behavior was helpful in setting modest goals for her treatment. Not many individuals like Jean stay in treatment long enough for a psychotherapist to really help. For caregivers in any setting, it is useful to know about such personality disorders so that they can set limited and reasonable goals for the care of their patients, even if the patients are with the caregivers only for a short time.

General Example 1

Individuals with narcissistic personality disorder provide much frustration to caregivers. With their selfish, demanding, and greedy nature, they are certainly no one's favorite. Individuals with narcissistic personality disorder have a sense of entitlement; they expect others to do things for them and do not want to be responsible for anything. Although they may not express it outright, their actions say, What have you done for me lately? They continue to have this attitude, even when others really may have gone out of their way. What can caregivers do for narcissistic individuals?

Kind and gentle ways that go far in helping many individuals with other personality disorders simply do not work when dealing with narcissistic persons. They do not understand kindness and do not respect it. In fact, they often will take advantage of the kind person and be more demanding and abrasive. Caregivers must not fall into the trap of constantly giving to these persons. Giving is not appreciated, and caregivers can become increasingly frustrated by the negative feedback of the encounter.

Caregivers must use a different approach with these individuals—in a word, *firmness*. You must set definite limits and strict rules for cooperation and make it clear what you are willing to do and not do in any given situation. Only by handling narcissistic individuals with firmness will you come out of the encounter with a positive feeling rather than feeling that these individuals have taken advantage of you.

General Example 2

Individuals with dependent personality disorder create problems for others. They do not want to take responsibility for their actions but rely on others to do most things for them. Such individuals feel comfortable around those who are giving. Eventually, those who spend most of their lives giving to others become tired of dependent persons, tired of the helping, feeding, and assisting that are required.

How can caregivers best deal with dependent persons? After you become aware that this personality disorder is the problem, gradually demand that some tasks, however small, be done by the dependent individuals. Attempting to change those who have dependent personality disorder to become fully responsible is not effective, but dependent persons can be forced to do some things. By doing so, you provide a degree of self-esteem that will in turn encourage dependent individuals to help themselves more than they had been doing previously.

Try making a contract with a dependent person. The contract could be stated or written formally. For example, you might say, "If you do this or that part, I will help you do the rest," or "When you finish doing what I expect of you, I will then do the following for you." It works. Both you and the other person will feel better about the interaction if there is at least minimal cooperation by the dependent person.

General Example 3

Suppose you are working with individuals who have histrionic personality disorder. As the caregiver, it is helpful to be aware of several facts. When histrionic persons become excited and overreact to events, it is useful to listen and quietly reassure them that everything is under control. Histrionic individuals respond well to quiet reassurance and support; however, it is important that this reassurance be done in private. Those with histrionic personality disorder love a crowd. People have a way of keeping histrionic persons stirred; therefore, if you want to calm down histrionic individuals who are overreacting, remove them from others and find a quiet place to do your reassuring.

If you want histrionic persons to remember your advice, write it down. In the excitement of the moment, histrionic individuals certainly will forget your sage advice and counsel. Writing a note about what you want these individuals to remember is useful. Also, if you must be away from those you are helping, a telephone call greatly reinforces any written messages that you have left.

As a caregiver, should you be a chameleon and adapt yourself to every different type of personality? Of course not, but altering your *style* somewhat, when it is necessary, can be useful in your caregiving. Whether you are a physician, nurse, aide, relative, friend, or any other caregiver, it makes your life easier and your work more effective if you consider what personality disorders you are encountering. Kindness and gentleness work wonders for those who have some personality disorders, whereas firmness and insistence are helpful for individuals who have other disorders. Even anger sometimes has a place in caregiving. Anger can be an expression of caring, especially in situations where persons are abusing your good intentions. When the individuals you are attempting to assist are utterly exasperating, expressing your anger without overreacting may be helpful. Your anger often will end the frustration of the moment and engender more cooperation. You will never change the basic personality of individuals with whom you are dealing, but you can alter the behavior in small but important ways so that you can be a more effective, competent caregiver. Although they are difficult to help, people with personality disorders can be rewarding to work with if you have patience and try to understand the nature of their disorders.

CHAPTER 13

UNUSUAL PSYCHIATRIC DISORDERS

The disorders I have grouped together in this chapter are interesting but not common. The first group is called the factitious disorders and the second is impulse-control disorders.

Factitious Disorders

Factitious disorders occur with physical symptoms or with psychological symptoms.

Factitious Disorder With Physical Symptoms

Factitious disorder with physical symptoms is called Munchausen syndrome, which is a rare disturbance. For not-so-obvious reasons, individuals with Munchausen syndrome have physical symptoms for which they request medical treatment, hospitalization, or even surgery, when none of these are warranted. However, these people are able to convince medical personnel that care is needed.

Individuals who are prone to Munchausen syndrome often have some experience in the medical field; they may be nurses, physicians, or technicians or other support personnel. Their familiarity with the medical system enables them to manipulate and obtain services that they want. There is some evidence that these individuals have suffered a form of childhood deprivation or have been rejected by one or both parents. They see in the physician or other health care worker a source of gratification for these formerly unmet needs for dependency and love. Some have a severely ill family member with whom they identify. Oddly enough, the wish to be cared for by these medical means is not really gratified because most medical caregivers eventually reject patients who have this disorder.

Individuals with Munchausen syndrome assume the role of patient and go to the physician or hospital with symptoms that appear to represent one or more diseases. The complaints are convincing or at least plausible to the medical caregiver. As a result, the patients are examined, tested, and diagnosed extensively. They sometimes become surgical patients and undergo an unusual number of operations. The illness appears to be under voluntary control and involves denial, lying, and manipulation, even though the patients may not admit any control over the illness.

There also is a compulsive component to the behavior. Individuals with this disorder move from one medical setting to another seeking to assume the role of patient. They frustrate the medical caregivers, who then refuse to treat them. When refused treatment, individuals with Munchausen syndrome move on to another place and repeat the behavior.

Factitious Disorder With Psychological Symptoms

In factitious disorder with psychological symptoms, the individuals have symptoms of emotional or mental illness. They seek treatment for their "illness" and often request admission to a psychiatric hospital. Symptoms may include psychotic behavior and simulated organic symptoms such as memory loss, disorientation, and confusion. Sometimes they give approximate answers to questions. For example, when asked to add 2 and 2, persons with this disorder may answer 5. The disorder may be easily confused with malingering. The reasons for assuming the role of a psychiatric patient are probably similar to those given by individuals who have Munchausen syndrome.

There is no standard treatment for factitious disorder with psychological symptoms. If a patient with Munchausen syndrome had symptoms of other disorders, these could be treated by the usual methods and perhaps some inroads could be made with the factitious disorders. I have no experience with these maladies because they are rare.

Impulse-Control Disorders

Everyone can be impulsive at times, but there are persons who have considerable trouble avoiding impulsive acts, even those that may be antisocial. These acts are generally harmful to the individuals. Among the impulse-control disorders are pathological gambling, pyromania (compulsive fire setting), kleptomania (compulsive stealing), and intermittent explosive disorder.

All of these disorders have several factors in common. Persons with impulse-control disorders seem unable to resist the impulse to do things that are harmful either to themselves or others. Before going through with the impulsive behavior, these individuals experience an increase in tension that is gradually relieved after the act. There also is a pleasurable feeling that accompanies the experience. Following the impulsive act, however, the individuals may feel guilt or remorse or may become self-critical. The cause of these behaviors is not well understood. At times, these disorders can be associated with organic brain disease or the use of drugs and alcohol. However, even if one of these problems is not the cause, the behaviors still occur in some people.

Generally, individuals have superego controls that prevent unusual behaviors. Because the results of these behaviors are often punishments, including long jail terms or huge debts, it is puzzling why people go through with the acts even when they may be aware of the consequences of those acts. The temporary feeling of pleasure and the relief of tension or psychic pain seem to overcome conscious thoughts about consequences.

Pathological Gambling

Case Example

Joe, age 40, was sent for consultation by his family for his excessive gambling. His desire to gamble started when he was an adolescent. At that time, he gambled on football and baseball games in the betting pools at school. As time went on, Joe bet on horses and then became a regular at Atlantic City casinos. A few years before I saw him, he had been working steadily in a middle-management office job. Joe was married and had two children. His persistent gambling resulted in his losing all moneys in his bank account. He then went to loan sharks, confident that he would be able to win big the next time. Occasionally, he did win, but he was always tempted to win even bigger. On several occasions when Joe was in debt, his parents bailed him out "to give him another chance." However, these attempts at rescuing him from his compulsive gambling were to no avail. There were times when Joe seemed to have a hold on himself. For several months, he worked steadily, put his money in the bank, paid his bills, and was a responsible father and husband. But then the gambling began again. Finally, his wife and children left him and went to live with his in-laws. Joe was destitute; an added complication was the threats on his life by loan sharks.

It was clear that Joe had hit bottom; he had no farther to go. He had no money, he was deeply in debt, and everyone but his parents had deserted him. After hearing his story, and ruling out organic illness and knowing the compulsive nature of his disorder, I referred him to Gamblers Anonymous (GA). This group's work is based on the model of Alcoholics Anonymous (AA); the group treats its members in the same way as AA does. In my opinion, attending GA is the best method for dealing with this pathological compulsion. Psychotherapy alone is not an effective method of treatment, but in conjunction with GA, there is hope for the compulsive gambler.

Joe accepted his disorder and went to GA. He continued in psychotherapy with me for a short time and did well. For his success, I have to give most of the credit to Joe for his attending GA.

Pyromania

Pyromania involves the compulsive urge to set fires, even if it means destroying property and injuring or killing people. As I write this chapter, the last of the severe fires on the California coast is being put out. There have been three deaths reported and more than 1,000 homes destroyed. It has been established that the fires were started by an arsonist.

Persons who set fires experience a thrill from witnessing the fire, and a relief of tension occurs. The diagnosis of pyromania is not made when individuals have schizophrenia, an organic illness, a conduct disorder of childhood, or antisocial personality disorder. More males than females have the impulse-control disorder pyromania.

Many theories have been advanced for the compulsion to set fires. None of the theories have been accepted as fundamentally true. Freud and others thought fire represented the sexual act, but this theory is not convincing. Another theory associates fire with feelings of anger, rage, betrayal, injustice, or inferiority.

Studies involving fire setters have uncovered some interesting facts. Most fire setters appear to lead normal everyday lives. Some have compulsions to set fires every night, whereas others do so sporadically. Some fire setters are volunteer fire fighters. The desire for power seems to be a motivating force for some fire setters. Other fire setters are more concerned with issues of control (i.e., putting out the fire) rather than the actual fire itself.

Few treatments have been tried for pyromania because fire setters have little motivation for treatment and seldom go to psychiatrists for help. When apprehended, they often end up in penal institutions.

Kleptomania

Persons with kleptomania steal for the pleasure derived from the act itself; there is little remorse or guilt. These individuals usually have sufficient money and do not need the items they steal. They may give the items away or hide them. The disorder appears to be more common among women.

There are many theories about why compulsive stealing occurs.

It is my impression that there is considerable aggression involved in this disorder. In patients whom I have treated, the idea of taking something away from a store or place of employment seemed to give them pleasure. Outsmarting the authorities, getting away with something, and unconsciously expressing anger may be motivations for kleptomania. Some theorize that the act has sexual implications.

Kleptomania usually begins in childhood or adolescence. Most cases do not come to the attention of mental health professionals until the patient has been apprehended. If the patient is motivated, psychotherapy and behavior therapy have been reported as successful in treating kleptomania.

Intermittent Explosive Disorder

Individuals with intermittent explosive disorder have a sudden onset of aggressive impulses that are out of proportion to any events going on at the time of the aggressive behavior. The act may result in the destruction of property or may be an assault on one or more persons. The disorder comes on and disappears suddenly. It occurs in persons who are normally not aggressive or explosive in between episodes.

Brain lesions such as those occurring in epilepsy have been implicated in this disorder. Most patients have a history of early trauma at birth or thereafter. Hyperactivity and encephalitis may be present in the patient's background.

Intermittent explosive disorder occurs more frequently in men, often in those who feel impotent but are also dependent on others in their environment. The disorder may be most evident in adolescence and the next decade of life, but as individuals mature and enter middle age, the disorder may gradually subside. Because of the dramatic nature of the disorder, patients often have poor work records and difficult marriages. Legal problems are common.

Treatment for intermittent explosive disorder is not clearly defined. Medications are sometimes helpful. If patients have depression or anxiety, treatment of these symptoms may help. Psychotherapy should be tried to eliminate possible underlying causes of anger.

What Can Families, Friends, and Caregivers Do?

Among the disorders described in this chapter, only pyromania and the factitious disorders cannot be successfully treated. The rest can be treated to some extent by psychotherapy and medication. Relatives and friends can report fire setters to authorities to prevent harm to people or property. Hospitals and physicians can be informed if family members or friends of the patients have evidence of any factitious disorder; beyond providing this information, little can be done for these patients.

Caregivers can be helpful to individuals who have any of the other impulse-control disorders. In cases of pathological gambling, families, friends, and caregivers must be aware of being enablers to the patients, thus allowing them to continue their behavior. Joe, for example, probably would have received treatment sooner if his parents had not rescued him financially and given him another chance. By doing so, they became enablers. As with alcoholic patients, enabling can delay acquiring the necessary help.

Although kleptomania usually comes to the attention of the family via complaints to police, the disorder is quite amenable to treatment. The family must take a therapeutic rather than a punitive approach to the problem. Proper psychotherapy should be obtained and may require that the family be involved in treatment along with the patient, since the reason for the stealing is usually found in the family dynamics.

When relatives or friends of individuals with intermittent explosive disorder become aware of frequent and sudden attacks of violence, they should seek an evaluation and therapy for these individuals from a psychiatrist. Physical causes of intermittent explosive disorder must first be ruled out, and medication may be required to control the violence. While attempting to be understanding of the problem, caregivers should firmly insist that treatment be obtained for the patients' welfare as well as their own. Caregivers may insist that the patients live elsewhere or that the police be called if these patients do not agree to treatment. As with other disorders, caregivers can be of enormous assistance to good psychiatric and psychological care of patients with intermittent explosive disorder.

PART III

MENTAL ILLNESS: THE PSYCHOSES

CHAPTER 14

MOOD DISORDERS: DEPRESSION AND MANIC STATES

Everyone has bad moods now and then. They may last a few hours, days, or even weeks. If they are not severe, most of us wait for our moods to go away. Moods usually wear off, and we return to our old happy, contented, thoughtful, or cynical self, depending on our basic personality. But if the mood lingers too long or is too far from our normal range of feelings, it becomes distressing. The mood can deepen to what psychiatrists call a clinical depression or be elevated to a mania.

How can a person tell the difference between a low mood and a significant depression? Anyone can tell whether the depression is due to just a bad day or is a deep depression that obviously needs treatment. But if a lowered mood lasts for several weeks and is clearly in response to a problem that the person has, it is quite likely to lift when the problem is solved. Some bad moods come on when there is no obvious external problem causing the change; such moods may lift spontaneously. However, whether the person has a low mood or significant depression, the depressed mood may become a clinical depression.

Generally, if a depressed mood goes on for weeks or seriously interferes with a person's functioning, the person needs professional help. I know one woman who endured a severe depression for 2 years. She thought of suicide on a number of occasions but did not seek help. Being religious, she said she tried to "pray my way out of it." Anyone can admire her courage and her will to work out the problem herself, but had she sought out treatment earlier, she would have been free of the depression after several months. In addition, as a self-employed worker, she had to give up many months of employment and salary, all of which could have been avoided.

I began practicing psychiatry just before the time antidepressant medication first became available. Depressive syndromes, which practitioners saw at that time, typically lasted at least several months and were known to go on for as long as 1 year. In unusual situations, depression lasted for years; however, most depressions were time limited, and eventually the patients recovered. In the meantime, the agony and pain of depression had to be endured. Patients have told me that severe depression is the most difficult experience that they have ever encountered, worse than any physical pain.

How can friends or family identify a serious depression? The individual's mood and energy level are low; there is little desire to do anything. Even the things that were most enjoyed by the person in the past are of no interest to him or her. Appetite for food disappears, and the individual eats to subsist, not because he or she wants to eat. There is little or no interest in sexual experiences. Sleep becomes difficult. Usually, depressed people have little trouble getting to sleep but they awaken early in the morning, sometimes at 1 or 2 A.M. Then, they cannot fall asleep again, and they lie awake obsessing about their problems and their inability to function. In this immobilized state, they often see suicide as the only way out of the severe pain that is experienced. In fact, most suicides are the result of depression. Caregivers, friends, and family members who observe depression in those to whom they are close should seek help as soon as possible so as to ward off the possibility of depression becoming worse, thus preventing suicide.

In contrast to those who have low moods and severe depression, some persons are subject to elevated moods. An elevated mood also may be of short duration or may last for months. The mood change may be mild and difficult to recognize from normal variations in mood. If the mood is elevated higher than is usual for someone, the individual may appear more energetic, work excessively long hours, and require little sleep. Psychiatrists speak of patients with this level of elevated mood as being *hypomanic*. Their condition may remain at this level, and aside from becoming irritable and impatient with others, they may get through this stage without incident. However, if the mood becomes more elevated and expansive, the patients lose their good judgment and do things that anyone can recognize as abnormal. When their mood reaches this level, the behavior of the patients is referred to as *manic*. For instance, a conscientious woman, while in a manic state, became impatient with a gasoline station attendant. She left the station without paying for the gas. A young man in a manic state "borrowed" a motorcycle that he saw in a parking lot and kept it for several days. Neither of these individuals would have used such poor judgment in their healthy mental state. Both of these patients were apprehended by the police, and family members brought them to me for treatment.

In full-blown manic states, the patients' behavior becomes grossly disturbed. Manic individuals are grandiose, feel they can do anything they wish, are often delusional, and may claim to have great influence or power. For example, a young man with little music ability told me he was a rock star; older persons can claim association with celebrities or well-known political figures. Some persons in manic states believe that they are well-known individuals, whereas others become paranoid and feel that people or organizations are against them. Patients who are manic do not realize that their behavior is abnormal. In these manic states, they are hard to control and often need the help of the police in order to be admitted to a hospital. Surprisingly, when patients receive the appropriate treatment in a hospital, these exaggerated manic states can be considerably improved in as little as 1 or 2 weeks.

The following discussions highlight some general information about clinical depression.

What Is the Frequency of Depression?

According to statistics from the National Institute of Mental Health, in the United States, about 9 million people suffer from one or more episodes of depression in a lifetime. Some estimates by experts place the number even higher—at about 15 million. This number includes those patients who suffer from organic mental disorders as well. Among the organic illnesses are hypothyroidism, brain tumors, endocrine disorders, and drug and alcohol abuse.

How Can Someone Recognize Depression?

In essence, clinical depression consists of a dramatic lowering of a person's mood. Clinical depression affects the individual mentally, physically, and psychologically. Anyone can recognize an individual who has a mild depression; he or she has fatigue, lack of energy, and mild sleep problems. Usually, these problems do not require any active treatment unless they recur and impede a person's functioning. If the depression deepens, the person becomes pessimistic and feels hopeless. Even small tasks that were easy to complete appear as huge hurdles. Interests that used to be enjoyable lose their luster. Appetite for food vanishes and sexual interest fades. Depressed persons have considerable trouble sleeping, usually in remaining asleep. Typically, they awaken at 1 or 2 A.M. and are not able to fall asleep for the rest of the night. During this time, there is little that depressed individuals do except ruminate about the terrible state of depression in which they find themselves. Some depressed individuals sleep excessively, but they are the exception. In daytime hours, there is an inability to concentrate. Because of their preoccupation with the lowered mood and the deep concern about how they feel, depressed persons do not remember recent events well. Guilt, worry, and agitation are often present. Sometimes the guilt reaches psychotic proportions. For example, a patient told me that his thoughts were evil and that by thinking bad thoughts he was influencing the health of a friend, causing him to become sick.

Along with the previously mentioned symptoms, many depressed people have extreme pessimism about the future and some develop suicidal thoughts. Attempts at suicide may occur, especially at certain stages of life. There are age-related peaks for suicide. The first occurs during late adolescence and young adulthood—roughly at ages 15–25 years. A second peak occurs at ages 45–55 years. The third peak in the suicide rate is seen among older persons, a group that has had a dramatic increase in suicides in recent years. This fact may be related to the increased aging population, with its accompanying loneliness, loss of function, and physical illness.

Most people who have clinical depression can be treated in the psychiatrist's office. After careful evaluation to rule out organic problems related to other diseases that require treatment, the patients often can benefit from antidepressant medication and psychotherapy. With such treatment, a partial improvement from the depression can be expected within several weeks. After several months, most patients are able to return to their normal level of functioning. In some cases, recovery requires a longer time. There also are some types of environmentally caused depressions that can be treated with psychotherapy alone, without the use of antidepressants. In the event of suicidal preoccupation, the therapist must evaluate whether the potential for suicide is imminent. If so, hospitalization usually is advisable; that is, the patients should be in a protected environment to prevent them from acting on suicidal ideas.

Two Types of Depression

For many years, mental health professionals have recognized that some depressions come on as the result of obvious external events such as the loss of a job or the death of a loved one. In these instances, it is assumed that the loss brought about the depression and that the symptoms are psychologically based. This type of depression has been called an *exogenous depression*. It usually occurs in individuals who are conscientious and perfectionist. When they suffer a loss of some kind, they become hurt and depressed, a so-called narcissistic injury.

In contrast, there are depressions that come on within days or weeks without any warning and with no obvious psychological cause. This type of depression is called an *endogenous depression*. It is caused by biological factors and is probably hereditary. Such mood disorders may be seen in parents, siblings, grandparents, uncles, aunts, and the extended family. This disorder formerly was called manic-depressive illness (now called bipolar disorder). Endogenous depression clinically resembles the exogenous form. The symptoms are identical, but those of endogenous depression may be more severe. Persons with endogenous depression speak of their experience of depression with surprise: "It came on right out of the blue." The depression may occur on a seasonal basis such as every spring or fall. In some instances, the depression may not recur for many years. These depressions are referred to by many as a "chemical imbalance" in the brain. The neurotransmitters in the brain that carry messages from one nerve cell to another are depleted. When this depletion occurs, the person is physically and mentally slowed down. The antidepressants that are currently available often can correct this chemical imbalance and help restore the individual to health.

Case Example 1: Exogenous Depression

One day, a new patient, Jim, came to my office. He was a 50-year-old married man who had a sudden onset of depression with markedly lowered feelings, sense of hopelessness about the future, and a general slowing down of physical activities (psychomotor retardation).

Jim had always been conscientious at his office job. He attended church regularly and thought of himself as a "good family man." Now he was unable to work and had lost interest in his former pastimes, such as bowling and reading. He had no trouble falling asleep, but upon awakening at 3 A.M., he was unable to resume sleeping. Suicide preoccupied Jim, especially at these early morning hours when he could not rid himself of his depressing thoughts. Jim had no history of psychiatric illness, and he had no family history of depression. Furthermore, Jim was referred by his internist, who could find no physical illness to account for his depression. I decided that in Jim's current mental state, it would be of no value to try to figure out the origin of his depression. When patients are extremely depressed, most are not able to think clearly enough to talk about the reasons for the depression. It is far more productive to delve into these issues when the patients have improved.

I decided to treat Jim with a combination of psychotherapy and antidepressant medication. I saw him twice a week in my office, as I concluded that he was not a serious suicide risk. After 2 weeks, Jim's sleep had improved, and he acknowledged that he had stopped regressing. His mood and appetite gradually improved. After about 4 weeks of treatment, Jim returned to work on a part-time basis. Two months later, he was considerably improved, and after 6 months, he was back to his normal level of functioning. Gradually, I reduced the medication and then stopped it entirely.

As Jim's mental state improved, I tried to ferret out the possible emotional and environmental reasons for his depression. As with many other patients who become depressed, Jim had difficulty expressing his emotions, especially his angry feelings. He usually related to his friends and co-workers in a mild and ingratiating manner, thus avoiding any hostility from them. Before his illness began, Jim was faced with a new boss, who was brusque, temperamental, and intimidating. Jim's natural way of dealing with people did not help him with the situation, and as a result, he became withdrawn and depressed.

Psychologically, Jim had problems with his angry impulses that were in conflict with his superego (conscience) desires. When faced with anger from others, he reacted with hurt feelings. Rather than deal directly with his anger by expressing it in an appropriate way, he held it in and turned it against himself.

In the course of psychotherapy with Jim, I tried to get him to deal with his passivity and help him with problems confronting people. We discussed his way of dealing with anger. His opinion was that as a religious person, it was sinful to be angry regardless of the circumstances. I tried to show him that anger had its uses and that if anger were used appropriately, it could be effective in helping him deal with people. Although he had considerable difficulty thinking about expressing any amount of anger and considering it

the "right" thing to do, he gradually understood the general principles of using emotions in the service of health.

It took about a year of psychotherapy before Jim was able to use
his emotions in ways that were good for him. He learned how to
handle his boss so that depression did not follow. He also developed a somewhat tougher skin so that criticism did not bother him
as much as it had previously.

Many patients do not wish to investigate the origins of their illness or understand the patterns that typically get them into trouble
emotionally. But for those who are able to take a hard look at themselves, insight into emotional problems, such as depression, can be
helpful in preventing future depression from returning.

After about a year of psychotherapy, and long after he had
stopped using medication, Jim was able to deal adequately and have
a working relationship with his boss that did not adversely affect him
in an emotionally distressing way.

During psychotherapy, the therapist helps the patient to gain insight into his or her typical patterns of behavior. By acting as an emotional "catalyst," the psychotherapist attempts to alter the patient's
former inadequate way of dealing with his or her environment. Furthermore, when the patient gains awareness about the etiology of his
or her illness, the patient often can prevent the recurrence of the
symptoms. The most valuable aspect of psychotherapy is not only
figuring out what causes pathology, but also preventing future illness
from occurring.

There are mood disorders that occur without any specific pre-
cipitating stress or psychological problem. The onset of the illness
may be sudden or gradual, but it seems to come out of the blue. There
may be some mild stressors at the time, but they play a minor role in
the illness or are incidental to the fact the mood alteration occurs.
These are the mood disorders that are hereditary and run in families.

Case Example 2: Endogenous Depression

Recently, I saw a 50-year-old executive who had been functioning
well. Gilbert was engaged in running a medium-size company. He
had felt competent and in control of his work. His family life was
in order, and he was enjoying a good relationship with his wife and

children. There were no pressing problems on his mind that he was not able to handle. But suddenly, Gilbert noticed that he was not able to sleep well; his complaint involved mostly early morning awakening. After a week of poor sleep, he became depressed, and small tasks began to look like mountains. Gilbert moved slowly, began procrastinating, and tended to forget things that ordinarily he would have no trouble remembering. Concentration became a severe problem. Within 2 weeks, he was completely unable to work. At home, he paced the floor and worried about his future. After another week of this inability to perform, Gilbert felt pessimistic about the future. At times, he thought of suicide as a way out, but he said that he thought he could never actually end his own life. He had a hard time believing that he could deteriorate to such a low level of functioning.

Inquiry into Gilbert's history revealed that he had experienced depression on two previous occasions. The first episode occurred in college, when he was jilted by a woman whom he had dated for 3 years. The second depression came on in the absence of any psychological problems, in much the same way as his current depression. In addition, I discovered that Gilbert's father and grandfather had depression. One of his uncle's had manic and depressed episodes (bipolar disorder).

After several weeks of treatment with an antidepressant, Gilbert felt somewhat improved, but it took many weeks before he was back to his usual self. Because his depressions were recurrent and he had a strong family history of mood disorders, I concluded that he had a biologically based illness. I decided that he should be on a maintenance dose of lithium to prevent depressions in the future. He readily accepted the recommendation.

I see Gilbert several times a year for evaluation and to check on his blood lithium level. Gilbert has been symptom free for about 10 years—a common story with patients who take lithium.

Classification of Mood Disorders

DSM-IV classifies the bipolar disorders and depressive disorders, which are briefly reviewed in the following discussions.

Bipolar Disorders

Mild forms of depression and "high" feelings are rather common to the general population. Such mood changes are transient and generally do not need expert help. These minor changes in mood are not included in the classification. Only the more severe forms of mood disorders are mentioned and discussed.

Bipolar I disorder.   Patients with bipolar I disorder have depression, manic periods, or both. When patients are depressed, their mood is low and they have all of the symptoms of depression described earlier in this chapter. When the patients have a manic episode, they become emotionally high, have an abnormal amount of energy, sleep and eat little, have grandiose ideas, and tend to go on wild spending sprees. If individuals with bipolar I disorder go untreated, their condition may eventually deteriorate into a psychotic state. Although environmental influences may play a part in bringing on the manic or depressed states, bipolar disorders are now known to be mostly hereditary.

Bipolar II disorder.   Patients with bipolar II disorder have recurrent major depressive episodes with hypomanic episodes (a mild form of mania). Bipolar disorders are further classified in DSM-IV according to the last alteration in mood (i.e., depressed, manic, mixed, or hypomanic).

Cyclothymic disorder.   Cyclothymic disorder can be viewed as a low-grade bipolar disorder; that is, both high and low moods occur. However, in comparison, the symptoms of cyclothymic disorder are milder than those of bipolar disorder. When patients experience high moods, they are overactive, irritable, and somewhat arrogant and argumentative. They feel especially good and do not have much patience with others who do not share their high spirits. This elevated mood is referred to as hypomania. When these patients are depressed, the lowered mood is not as deep as in bipolar disorder, but it can be disturbing to some patients and can last for many months.

Bipolar disorder not otherwise specified.   If a patient has symptoms that do not clearly fit the bipolar disorders classification but are atypical, then the disorder is labeled bipolar disorder not otherwise specified.

Three other mood disorders classified in DSM-IV are 1) mood disorder due to a general medical condition, 2) substance-induced mood disorder, and 3) mood disorder not otherwise specified.

Depressive Disorders

Major depressive disorder.   Major depressive disorder is a severe form of depression. It may appear as a single depression, or it may recur a number of times in a person's life. This type of depression may be brought on by emotional and environmental factors (exogenous), or it may be a biological (endogenous) form.

Dysthymic disorder (formerly called depressive neurosis).   Dysthymic disorder is a mild to moderate type of depression and has to occur over a period of at least 2 years. The basis for the depression is presumed to be psychological conflicts, which cause the person to become depressed.

Depressive disorder not otherwise specified.   A depression that does not meet the criteria for any of the depressive disorders classified in DSM-IV is considered a depressive disorder not otherwise specified. An example of a depressive disorder not otherwise specified is seasonal affective disorder. The cause of this depression is the lack of light that occurs in the late fall and winter seasons. Patients with this problem respond well to the daily use of artificial light during the winter season.

Manic Attacks:
The Other Side of Depression

Some persons with bipolar disorder suffer from manic attacks only. Others cycle through both the manic and depressed phases. Although I have described manic episodes earlier in this chapter, an example of this behavior will better illustrate how such episodes can be recognized.

Case Example

A 30-year-old woman, Ann, was brought to the emergency room for treatment. She was very loud and talkative. She jumped around from one subject to another. She displayed an unusually high mood. I tried to find out what had happened to account for her condition, but she was unable to tell me about it with any clarity. Fortunately, her mother was with her and gave the following information: Ann was working as an office manager and had been employed at the same place for 5 years. Recently, she broke up with her male friend, whom she had been seeing for several years. At first, she was markedly upset and depressed. Then, she gradually improved but began behaving strangely. She had overcharged her credit card by $2,000 and had purchased a new car without having sufficient funds to maintain monthly payments. Ann had told everyone that she felt fine and that nothing was wrong. In addition, she seldom slept and cared little about eating. Ann made many calls to friends, some of whom called her mother to ask what was wrong with her. She could not control her emotions and when confronted by her family about her behavior, she began to suspect that they were going to harm her. When this occurred, her parents decided that she needed to be examined by a psychiatrist.

Ann was difficult to interview. It was apparent that she was in a manic state and needed to be treated. She was too ill to be treated as an outpatient, so after much persuasion, she agreed to be admitted to the hospital. While there, I gave her a major tranquilizer and lithium to help her mood return to normal. After about 1 week with the medication and the calming effect of the treatment team in the hospital, she was much improved. After another week, Ann was sent home and was asked to continue treatment at my office. Ann took a maintenance dose of lithium while going to psychotherapy weekly.

Although rejection by her lover appeared to be the event that precipitated Ann's illness, it was not the single cause of her sudden problem. Bipolar disorder is an inherited illness that usually runs in families. In fact, I learned that her father and an aunt had a history of bipolar disorder as well. Unlike patients who have other disorders, and despite the severity of the symptoms involved, patients who have bipolar disorder do not readily accept the fact that they have a mental illness that is likely to recur. It usually takes two or three serious hospitalizations to convince them of the true nature of the disorder, at which time patients are much more likely to conform to treatment with medications. Patients who are well controlled on drugs do not need to be seen frequently, perhaps only once every 2–3 months.

Lithium carbonate (Eskalith, Lithobid) has been used successfully in the treatment of bipolar disorder in preventing or at least reducing the severity of both the manic and the depressive phases of this illness. It also has been useful in reducing the recurrence and severity of major depressive disorder. The result has been a savings of billions of health care dollars in terms of fewer hospitalizations and the early return of patients to their previous occupations.

More recently, two other medications have been used for bipolar disorder when lithium is not helpful or the patient has kidney disease. These are Tegretol (carbamazepine) and Depakote (divalproex sodium).

Medications for Mood Disorders

In 1957, the first antidepressant became available to psychiatrists for use in treating depression. Before that time, the only treatment procedure that was commonly in use was electroconvulsive therapy (ECT). ECT was helpful in treating both manic states and depression. Despite the negative view that the average person has about this type of therapy, ECT is still used in the treatment of depression when all else fails. ECT remains an effective treatment.

Currently, there are four groups of antidepressant medications: 1) the tricyclic antidepressants, 2) the monoamine oxidase inhibitors (MAOIs), 3) the selective serotonin reuptake inhibitors (SSRIs), and 4) a miscellaneous group of drugs.

Tricyclic Antidepressants

The first drug used for depression was imipramine; it was marketed with the trade name Tofranil. Although imipramine was the first drug in the group of tricyclic antidepressants, many others have followed. The commonly used tricyclic drugs include the following:

- Asendin (amoxapine)
- Aventyl, Pamelor (nortriptyline)
- Elavil (amitriptyline)
- Norpramin, Pertofrane (desipramine)
- Sinequan, Adapin (doxepin)
- Tofranil (imipramine)
- Vivactil (protriptyline)

The neurotransmitters in the brain are lowered in depression and elevated in manic states. These chemical messengers carry impulses from one nerve cell to another. They are regularly manufactured by the brain and then eliminated. The tricyclic drugs block the neurotransmitters from the normal cycle of "uptake" or elimination in the synapse. As a result, neurotransmitters rise to normal levels, with a corresponding improvement in depression. There are other theories about how antidepressant drugs work (for more detailed information, see *Kaplan and Sadock's Synopsis of Psychiatry*, Seventh Edition).

The main symptoms that are seen as side effects of tricyclic drugs are dry mouth, constipation, and swelling of the hands and feet. Some patients have difficulty with close vision, and certain types of glaucoma can become worse. A rapid heartbeat and palpitations are common. Inability to urinate and paralysis of the small intestine are side effects, although I have never had a patient with this latter problem. Rarely, tremor, weakness, and problems with motor coordination can occur. As with any drug, allergic reactions to tricyclic antidepressants are possible.

Lowering the dose of medication will reduce the side effects. Also, with a patient's increasing age, the side effects become worse. Therefore, lower doses are given to older persons.

Monoamine Oxidase Inhibitors

Among many other substances in the brain, monoamine oxidase is an enzyme that deactivates the neurotransmitters dopamine, norepinephrine, and serotonin; therefore, the activity of nerve transmission is slowed down. The medications known as MAOIs inhibit the action of monoamine oxidase, thus increasing activity in the synapse. If the level of neurotransmitters is low, as in clinical depression, the MAOIs will raise the level and restore the neuronal activity to normal.

Commonly used MAOIs include the following:

- Marplan (isocarboxazid)
- Nardil (phenelzine)
- Parnate (tranylcypromine)

The MAOIs have an interesting history. Their usefulness in the field of psychiatry was discovered by accident. When the scourge of tuberculosis was still prevalent in the 1940s and 1950s, a drug called iproniazid was used for treatment of the disease. At that time, most patients with tuberculosis were treated in large institutions. Many of the patients were depressed because of the prolonged illness and the isolation from friends and family. The physicians and nurses who were caring for these patients noted that many of those who received this drug for their tuberculosis improved emotionally as well; their depression improved. On further investigation into the mechanism of action of the drug, its antidepressant activity could be explained. After that, the drug was used for the treatment of clinical depression.

As usually happens, when one drug in a class of drugs is manufactured, other similar drugs are produced to compete with the first. Several new MAOI drugs were made available to physicians. After a few years of regular use, psychiatrists began to report that some patients receiving MAOIs had severe headaches and even strokes. A small number died as a result. Subsequent investigation into this phenomenon revealed that a substance, called tyramine, in certain foods in combination with the drug caused a large increase in blood pressure, which was responsible for the side effects. Tyramine is present in foods such as aged cheeses and meats and in beverages such as beer and wine. If patients refrain from eating foods and drinking beverages with tyramine, the high blood pressure does not occur, and the drug can be used safely.

The MAOIs are used when other antidepressants prove to be ineffective and for certain types of depression for which they are known to be especially helpful.

The most important side effect of MAOIs is high blood pressure, as mentioned previously, but this can be avoided easily with the proper diet. Many individuals experience postural hypotension when getting up quickly from a sitting or lying position. The blood pressure does not adapt rapidly enough to the change in position, and the patients experience light-headedness and may even faint. Other side effects include dry mouth, constipation, difficulty urinating, and sexual problems, such as delayed ejaculation and impotence. None of these side effects are common. Rare cases of liver damage also have been reported.

Selective Serotonin Reuptake Inhibitors

Only a few years ago, the first SSRIs were introduced to psychiatrists. These new drugs are considered better than the older antidepressants because of their effectiveness and because they have fewer side effects. They do not cause drowsiness or weight gain or have an adverse effect on the heart. In addition, the medications can be taken once a day, in contrast to multiple doses for the other antidepressants.

Among the new SSRIs are the following:

- Paxil (paroxetine)
- Prozac (fluoxetine)
- Zoloft (sertraline)

These medications begin to help depressed patients after about 2 weeks. Usually, in 4 weeks there is a noticeable improvement in symptoms. As with all antidepressants, 6–8 weeks are required for an adequate assessment of the drug. For active patients who are able to work despite their depression, these medications are especially useful. Among the common side effects are headaches, nausea, diarrhea, and dizziness.

Miscellaneous Drugs

Among the other antidepressant drugs are a miscellaneous group that includes Ludiomil (maprotiline) and Desyrel (trazodone). These are chemically different from the other drugs described. They have side effects that are similar to those of the tricyclic antidepressants.

Other Uses for Antidepressants

SSRIs have been shown to be helpful in the treatment of obsessive-compulsive disorder. The exact mechanism for this therapeutic reaction is not known.

Small doses of antidepressants can be helpful in the treatment of pain. If used along with traditional pain medication, they enable the patient to take lower doses of the pain pills while obtaining the same pain relief.

Another use of antidepressants is in the treatment of panic attacks associated with agoraphobia (fear of leaving home or other familiar places). For example, a small dose of Tofranil (imipramine) blocked the panic attacks of a 25-year-old female patient of mine. Instead of having to confine her traveling to local sites in a suburban town, she was able to drive long distances from home.

What Can Families, Friends, and Caregivers Do?

It is important for family and friends to be aware that all mood changes are not solely the result of life's experiences. There are biological and organic illnesses that cause changes in mood, as well as emotional and psychological reasons. It should be left to the internist or family practitioner to investigate any physical disorders. A psychiatrist can then evaluate and prescribe appropriate medications, if they are indicated.

I have heard relatives, friends, and caregivers speak of depressed persons as being lazy. It is true that depression does not lead to productivity, but clinically depressed individuals cannot get themselves going as well as others do. It is as though they are dragging a load behind them. There is a heaviness of body and spirit. Of course, caregivers should encourage depressed individuals to move their muscles and do small tasks, but the accusation of laziness is inappropriate. Assuming that patients are under the proper care, family members, friends, or caregivers can be helpful in motivating the patients to take small steps to help themselves. Encouragement and support are important to anyone who is depressed.

Depressed patients do not need lectures on how to live. They do not need to be told You have to have the guts to face life. But people with depression do need *firmness* from those around them. It helps to *structure* their day. Help patients do small things on schedule throughout the day. It is of no benefit to allow depressed patients to stay in bed late in the morning or to spend time in bed during the day. Staying in bed serves no useful purpose and prevents them from sleeping well at night.

Depressed persons often have an exaggerated sense of guilt. Caregivers should not try to talk them out of their guilt feelings but should listen attentively and assure patients that their feelings may change with time. Friends and family who listen are a great source of security to depressed persons.

If there is a preoccupation with suicide, this information should not be withheld from the therapist. If patients do not want their caregivers or friends to tell the psychiatrist about suicidal ideas, this request should *not* be honored. It just might be lifesaving to reveal these suicidal thoughts to the treating psychiatrist or psychotherapist.

In manic states, patients often are hard to control. Caregivers should attempt to be firm with manic patients. Firmness can be helpful at times; at other times, it may be necessary to get outside help from the police or a medical emergency squad, for example.

Once manic patients are under control after a period of hospitalization, the family or friends can do much to help patients conform to treatment by keeping their therapists' appointments and taking medications regularly.

Sometimes it is necessary for the whole family to be in treatment to help one person who is suffering from a mood disorder. At other times, it is useful to have one or two of the family members attend some of the therapy sessions. Information discussed in therapy can be used later to reinforce the patient's attitudes toward healthy ways of thinking.

CHAPTER 15

SCHIZOPHRENIC DISORDERS

chizophrenia usually begins at an early age, often in adolescence. That's when it started for Roger.

Case Example

Roger had an uneventful childhood. He was a quiet, studious young man who never gave his parents or teachers any trouble. The only concern that his parents had about him was his lack of interest in friends. Roger was a loner. He seldom brought anyone home and did not participate in the usual activities that interest boys. His parents encouraged him to join the Boy Scouts and team sports. Nothing that involved his peers seemed to interest him.

Roger became withdrawn. He talked only when spoken to but rarely offered any conversation at home. Then, one day his parents noted that he was in his room, staring into space. When asked what was troubling him, he did not respond. Roger had hidden all his valuables but did not say why he had done so. At times, he appeared to turn his head in a certain direction, as if listening to someone in the room. But no one was there. Occasionally, he uttered some words that made little sense. A strange mood accompanied his actions. He often smiled inappropriately without talking. He was not overtly upset but appeared to be more in a dream world. His behavior was unusual and quite frightening to his parents.

When I first saw Roger, his behavior had changed little. He said a few things, such as "It's a trick. I have to watch out for them. They're after me." When asked who it was that was after him, he did not respond. Even in my presence, he appeared to be hearing voices—auditory hallucinations.

Roger was too acutely ill to be treated as an outpatient. I was concerned about his safety. I recommended that he be hospitalized in a psychiatric unit of a general hospital for a period of several weeks. His parents agreed, and treatment began. I found out that his condition did not begin abruptly; rather, he had become increasingly withdrawn and had been acting strangely for some months. His parents felt he was alone too much and was studying too hard. They had been kind to him and had hoped that his symptoms would go away, but instead they grew worse.

Upon admission to the hospital, it became apparent that Roger had a schizophrenic disorder. I prescribed antipsychotic medication and saw him daily for psychotherapy. I and the social worker talked with his parents, while the nurses talked with Roger individually and in group therapy. After 1 week, he improved slightly. The disturbing hallucinations diminished, and he became less withdrawn. By the second week, he began talking more, but he had few emotional reactions to things. After several weeks, he was discharged to a day hospital, where treatment was continued for a few more months. However, he was not able to return to school. He never regained his former personality or level of functioning, and he appeared to remain in a somewhat debilitated state. I continued to see Roger periodically in my office for medication maintenance and psychotherapy and encouraged him to go to the local community mental health center. His prognosis was quite poor.

Unfortunately, a significant number of patients like Roger who develop schizophrenia do not return to their former levels of functioning with our current treatment methods.

What Is Schizophrenia?

Schizophrenia has many forms and may not be one disorder. It is a mental illness that affects thinking, feeling, and behavior.

In schizophrenia, there is a "splitting" that occurs in the mind. It is not a split personality, as is commonly thought, but a splitting in the functioning of the mind. Logical thought and the ability to feel emotions are frequently impaired, but the ability to calculate and remain oriented to time, place, and person remains intact. For example, Roger was able to do simple math problems, even at the height of his illness. He knew where he was and was well oriented as to time, although he had auditory hallucinations. Furthermore, his thinking was paranoid and his bland feelings were inappropriate to what was happening to him. Psychiatrists call these bland feelings *flattened affect*.

A prominent symptom of schizophrenia is a thought disorder. The person's logical thought patterns break down, and the associations that he or she makes are loose. For example, a patient may be talking about one topic and quickly go to another without any apparent connection. In severe forms of schizophrenia, the connections between thoughts and words are so bizarre that the condition is called *word salad*.

Logical thought also may be based on a false belief. For example, if a schizophrenic patient believes his or her food is poisoned, he or she will do everything to avoid the food. It might even include going on a hunger strike, which would be a logical thing to do if the patient believed the food was poisoned. Thus, there is no problem in logic, but the patient's basic beliefs are abnormal, and his or her responses and behavior are in keeping with the false beliefs.

Among the other symptoms of schizophrenia are behaviors such as mutism (i.e., the person does not speak at all). Peculiar mannerisms and stereotypical movements also are common. Regression to childhood with wetting and soiling can occur in severely ill patients.

Schizophrenia usually begins in adolescence or early adult life, but it can start even as late as middle age. As patients grow older, however, the severity of the symptoms tends to diminish somewhat. At ages 50–60 years or older, some patients appear to be relatively mentally healthy.

The course of schizophrenia mainly takes two forms. One is relatively acute, has a brief duration, and resolves quickly, with few if any aftereffects. This acute form is believed to be influenced more by the environment of the patient and less by hereditary or constitutional factors. The second form has a more insidious onset. The symptoms are less acute, but the patient is unable to function over long periods of time. There usually is deterioration in the person's overall behavior; the prognosis is poor. In the case example, Roger has this second type of schizophrenia. This second form of schizophrenia is believed to be caused more by hereditary and biological factors and less by the environment.

Patients with mental illness occupy about 25% of all hospital beds in the United States. Of these, schizophrenic patients represent the largest number. One of every 100 children born in the United States will, at some time during his or her life span, develop the illness. This number is remarkably high. Despite that schizophrenia affects so many people in our population, there is little understanding of the illness, and insufficient effort has been applied to researching the nature of the illness. Schizophrenia is extremely devastating to individuals and may immobilize them for life. The families of patients with schizophrenia endure considerable stress in trying to handle patients' recurring symptoms.

Origins of Schizophrenia

The whole story of the cause of schizophrenia is yet to be told. Researchers are pursuing the problem with increasing attention. Some facts are known. First of all, there is some good evidence that the disorder is at least partially hereditary. Schizophrenia occurs in about 1% of the population. But if one parent has schizophrenia, the children of that parent have a 10%–15% chance of having the illness. If both parents have schizophrenia, the chances are 30%–50%, depending on the research studies. These statistics occur regardless of whether the children are raised in the parental home or in foster homes. Also, if an identical twin develops schizophrenia, the other twin has a high probability of getting the illness—about 30%–50%. Although these facts do not prove that schizophrenia is inherited, they represent strong evidence that the illness occurs in families.

Do environmental factors play a part in causing schizophrenia? Perhaps. Many stressors have been identified as possible causative agents for the illness, although none have been proven to bring on or continue the process of schizophrenia. Not too many years ago, a heavy blame was placed on poor or inadequate mothering. It was believed that the mothers of schizophrenic patients did not communicate well with their children and regularly gave out double messages to them, thus causing gross confusion in the children's developing minds. This theory was largely speculative and did not stand up to solid research.

Other environmental factors such as poverty, poor education, overcrowding in cities, and vitamin deficiencies have been cited as causes. Although such influences may play a part in bringing on schizophrenia, it is difficult to prove true.

Types of Schizophrenia

DSM-IV lists five types of schizophrenia:

1. *Catatonic type.* The "stuporous" form of schizophrenia is characterized by withdrawal, little or no talking (mutism), and repeated stereotypical movements or postures. Patients may remain immobile for hours at a time and not respond to questions or comments. Some patients display a "waxy flexibility," which means that the patients' arms can be placed in various positions and will remain there for long periods of time.

   Another form of this disorder is "excited" catatonia. Excited catatonic patients suddenly become overactive and have purposeless movements. These patients also may become destructive and dangerous. Patients have been known to switch rapidly from one form of catatonic behavior to another. For example, quiet, immobile, and mute patients may suddenly fly into a rage and hit someone. Others may go through a destructive wild stage and quickly become immobile and mute.

2. *Paranoid type.* The paranoid type of schizophrenia is one of

the better-known forms of mental illness. Patients who are paranoid are suspicious and distrustful and have delusions (false beliefs not usually found in the patients' culture). The patients may believe that someone on radio or TV is speaking directly to them or referring to them. They may believe that the Federal Bureau of Investigation (FBI) or police are trailing them or bugging their telephones. Sometimes, the patients may feel that another person is putting thoughts in their minds, or they may think that they have the ability to place thoughts in someone else's mind.

Although the patients have disturbances in their beliefs, the patients' feelings are usually appropriate to what they are thinking. For example, if they think that someone is after them, they may be appropriately fearful. In addition, paranoid schizophrenic patients often can be reasonable about matters that do not concern their specific paranoia.

3. *Disorganized type.*   After a gradual onset of the disorganized type of schizophrenia, the behavior of patients becomes inappropriate. They may laugh frequently and become silly. Because of a marked disorder in thinking, the patients are hard to understand. They have great difficulty expressing logical thoughts. They may make up new words (neologisms) that have meaning only to them. Hallucinations and delusions are often present. This form of schizophrenia is quite severe, and patients who suffer from it seldom get completely well, even with the new antipsychotic medications.

4. *Undifferentiated type.*   The undifferentiated type is a mixture of symptoms and is one of the most common manifestations of schizophrenia. Hallucinations and delusions are common, and some disturbance in logical thinking can occur. The affect (feelings) is dull or flat. After several attacks of acute symptoms of schizophrenia, the patients may gradually develop this undifferentiated form of the illness.

5. *Residual type.*   After the acute symptoms of schizophrenia subside and patients are functioning to some degree, they may be diagnosed as having the residual type. But even if patients have this type of schizophrenia, some symptoms remain. Some

social withdrawal, poor work performance, a flattened affect, and a mild thought disorder may be present.

Is Schizophrenia a Modern Illness?

There is evidence that schizophrenia existed in biblical times and has been present throughout history in one form or another. Ancient cultures regarded the mentally ill as possessed by the devil or involved with witchcraft. However, in some older cultures, mentally ill persons were considered saints, which is true even today in countries that are more primitive.

In the 18th century, a French physician, Philippe Pinel, removed mentally ill patients from the dungeons where they were routinely kept and moved them to settings that were more suitable for their care. This change represented the beginning of more humane care for the mentally ill.

Later, during the early part of the 19th century, Benjamin Rush, a physician in Philadelphia, treated mentally ill patients in a hospital setting. In a book he wrote on the subject of treatment, he described mental illness well, but care included cold-water baths and bloodletting, which were popular at the time.

In later years, Dorothea Dix and others did much to encourage the creation of hospitals for the mentally ill throughout the United States. More recently, with the advent of new medications, the mental health movement has encouraged discharging patients from large psychiatric institutions to local community hospitals or community mental health centers.

Recently, there has been significant progress in the treatment of the severely mentally ill, of which patients with schizophrenia compose the largest group. With the introduction of medications for patients with psychoses, a radical change in the practice of psychiatry occurred. In 1954, Dr. Nathan Kline, a researcher at Rockland State Hospital in Orangeburg, New York, described a drug that was useful in treating psychotic behavior. The drug was called reserpine. It was derived from a root and had been used for years in India for the treatment of high blood pressure and for sedation. When given to schizo-phrenic patients, it appeared to be of considerable value. Shortly thereafter, a new drug called Thorazine (chlorpromazine) was synthesized. It, too, had antipsychotic properties. These drugs were the beginning of medical treatment of the major psychoses. As a result of these developments and subsequent drug therapy, one-half of the hospitalized mentally ill population was eventually discharged to outpatient settings.

How Do Antipsychotic Drugs Work?

Drugs used in the treatment of the psychoses are referred to as *antipsychotics, neuroleptics,* or *major tranquilizers.* For the sake of simplicity, I use the term *antipsychotic drugs.* Most of the antipsychotic drugs are presumed to cause a change in the brain through their effects on certain neurotransmitters. In schizophrenia, there is an excess of the neurotransmitter dopamine. This excess causes changes in thinking, feeling, and behavior. When medications such as Thorazine (chlorpromazine) or Haldol (haloperidol) are used in these patients, the action of dopamine on receptors in the synapses is partially blocked. The transmission of impulses from one nerve cell to another is diminished, thus reducing the symptoms. The detailed mechanism of action of these drugs is probably much more complicated than this simple explanation; it is currently being studied by researchers.

Classification of Antipsychotic Medications

There are several chemical classes of drugs used in the treatment of schizophrenic patients and patients with other psychoses. The various chemical groups are significant only to the researcher.

In practice, it is important to the psychiatrist whether a medication is effective in treating symptoms and whether the side effects of the drugs are tolerable. The best medication is highly effective and has few bothersome side effects. Most of the current antipsychotic medications work about equally well, and the side effects differ only slightly. A psychiatrist may choose one drug over another because he or she has had more success with it or is more familiar with its use. The choice also may be determined by whether the patient is acutely ill or chronically ill and in a hospital or at home and able to work.

The following is a list of the more common antipsychotic drugs.

- Clozaril (clozapine)
- Haldol (haloperidol)
- Loxitane (loxapine)
- Mellaril (thioridazine)
- Moban (molindone)
- Navane (thiothixene)
- Risperdal (risperidone)
- Serentil (mesoridazine)
- Stelazine (trifluoperazine)
- Taractan (chlorprothixene)
- Thorazine (chlorpromazine)
- Trilafon (perphenazine)

Treatment With Antipsychotic Drugs

When antipsychotic drugs are used for schizophrenia or other psychoses, the acute symptoms of the disorder usually resolve in days or weeks. Symptoms such as delusions, hallucinations, paranoid ideas, and odd behaviors are often brought under control within a short period. In some instances, more time is needed; in others, the symptoms may be decreased but remain chronic. In general, the more acute and sudden the onset of schizophrenia, the more likely the symptoms will resolve quickly. By contrast, when the symptoms come on slowly and over a long time, medications to treat the illness are less effective.

In addition, when patients have severe withdrawal and a flat affect (little expressed feeling), they may not respond well to the standard antipsychotic drugs. These negative symptoms of schizophrenia are extremely resistant to change. However, one of the drugs in the aforementioned list, Clozaril (clozapine), has been effective with patients showing negative symptoms. However, this drug has one serious side effect—a drop in the white blood cell count, which is called *agranulocytosis*. To prevent this complication, patients' blood has to be monitored weekly. If the white blood cell count drops too low, the medication must be stopped.

Side Effects of Antipsychotic Drugs

There are a number of common side effects of antipsychotic drugs that are not dangerous. The side effects include symptoms such as skin rash, dryness of the mouth, constipation, and allergy to the medications. A serious side effect is inflammation of the liver, or *hepatitis*. Most of these side effects disappear if the medication is stopped.

The majority of the bothersome side effects of the antipsychotic drugs involve the nerve cells of the brain that have to do with muscle movement. The so-called extrapyramidal system of the brain is affected. This system is responsible for the smooth movement of voluntary muscle. The antipsychotic drugs interfere with the proper coordination of the movements. As a result, the following six symptoms may occur:

1. *Akinesia* is a limitation in the movements of the arms and legs while walking and a partial loss of facial expression.
2. *Akathisia* is a restlessness of the muscles. The patient is unable to sit still and often gets up, paces, and wrings the hands.
3. *Dystonia* is an abnormality in muscle tone, resulting in spasm of muscles of the neck, eyes, jaws, or larynx. The spasms come on suddenly and can be frightening. Fortunately, this side effect is uncommon.

4. *Pseudoparkinsonism* is a syndrome that resembles Parkinson's disease in older patients. Hand tremors, muscle weakness, and stiffness occur. The patient leans forward when walking, takes short steps, and sometimes has difficulty stopping. The patient does not swing his or her arms but holds them stiffly at his or her side. Jerking of the arms and legs also may occur.
5. *Tardive dyskinesia* is a serious side effect of the prolonged use of antipsychotic drugs. It occurs in 20%–40% of patients after they have been on the medications for years. Tardive dyskinesia includes involuntary movements of the lips, facial tics, abnormal chewing movements, and protrusion of the tongue. These symptoms can be distressing to the patients and quite distracting to observers. When the antipsychotic drugs are stopped, the symptoms do not necessarily go away. The longer these drugs are used and the higher the dose, the more likely symptoms will occur. Currently, there is no remedy for this condition, but research is being done to find a solution to this disabling side effect.
6. *Neuroleptic malignant syndrome* is a serious complication that may occur when high doses of antipsychotic medication are prescribed in a hospital setting. The syndrome includes fever, muscle rigidity, irregular heart rate, and severe perspiration; in some cases, death has resulted. Once diagnosed, neuroleptic malignant syndrome is quite treatable by discontinuing the medication and giving supportive treatment. But if the syndrome is unrecognized, it can be dangerous.

In general, the side effects of antipsychotic medications can be altered in the following ways:

- Some patients can develop tolerance for the drugs after they have been taking them for several weeks.
- The psychiatrist can reduce the dosage and minimize the side effects.
- An alternative antipsychotic medication can be substituted for the first one.
- Drugs to counter the side effects can be used. These are so-

called anticholinergic drugs, such as Cogentin (benztropine), Artane (trihexyphenidyl), and the antihistamine Benadryl (diphenhydramine). Although helpful in reducing side effects, these medications do not eliminate all the troubling symptoms of the antipsychotic drugs.

Using Antipsychotic Medication for Schizophrenia

Case Example

Some time ago, I was asked to evaluate a 21-year-old man named Tom. His family reported that he had been acting strangely for about 2 months. Tom was attending a local college. Lately, he was spending an excessive amount of time in his room. When his mother went to inquire what he was doing, Tom could not really give her a definitive answer. He seemed vague and uncertain. She noticed that he appeared to stare a lot. When asked what he was thinking about, Tom could not answer. He also had little interest in contacting the few friends that he had. Then, one day Tom suddenly blurted out that he could not take it any longer: "These guys are not going to get me. They've been following me for a long time. They want information." When asked who was following him, Tom was uncertain. He made references to the FBI and the police. He said that he heard messages on the radio and on TV that bothered him. His parents reported that Tom also seemed to be listening to something when there was no one around but his mother. Yet, Tom continued to do homework and he attempted to go to school. Finally, he became so distraught that he had to stay home. His parents realized that he was suffering from a mental illness. They decided to take Tom for an evaluation.

When Tom entered my office, he appeared frightened and withdrawn. Although he did not speak much, it was apparent to me that he was grossly paranoid and was having auditory hallucinations. He appeared to be in an acute psychotic state and needed immediate help. I recommended that he be admitted to a local hospital that had a psychiatric unit. Tom resisted the idea, but after a while, his parents and I persuaded him to go.

Tom was suffering from an acute schizophrenic disorder. In considering this diagnosis, I had to confirm with Tom and his parents that Tom was not using street drugs because these can cause similar symptoms.

After a few days in the hospital, Tom felt somewhat better. I gave him an antipsychotic drug, Haldol (haloperidol). Within 1 week, most of his acute symptoms had subsided. Some of his paranoid ideas and fears took longer to treat. The nursing staff and I held individual sessions with him, and he also attended group meetings. His recovery went well, except for some annoying side effects from the medication. After 3 weeks in the hospital, Tom was sent home and he soon returned to school. I followed up with him in my office for a 6-month period on a weekly basis. After that, I saw him monthly for another 6 months.

One year after the onset of his illness, Tom appeared completely recovered. I made no attempt to find any underlying cause for his mental disturbance other than the obvious: his need for more socializing and less time spent exclusively on schoolwork and more on recreation.

In contrast to popular belief, psychiatrists do not psychoanalyze patients with psychotic disorders. Psychoanalysis was attempted by competent psychiatrists before antipsychotic medications were commonly used. The analysis took years to complete, and the results, with an occasional exception, were disappointing. I recommend the autobiographical account of Joanne Greenberg, *I Never Promised You a Rose Garden,* for those interested in reading more about the long-term treatment of schizophrenia. Her story later became a popular movie.

With the current treatment methods, patients like Tom can expect to return to work or school in 1–3 months from the onset of treatment.

Do patients like Tom suffer relapses? The answer is yes, some do. But many patients have only one episode of mental illness in their entire lives. However, if a relapse of schizophrenia occurs, it is treated in much the same way, usually in a hospital. In addition, the patients take medications for a longer time, perhaps for 1–2 years.

There are many patients with schizophrenia who have a chronic form of the illness. They require long-term treatment with medication to maintain functional or semifunctional states. In such cases, attendance at a local community mental health center is valuable. Here, patients can attend individual and group sessions, as well as a day care center if needed.

One of the most effective tools to deal with the chronic forms of schizophrenia is education. In hospitals, clinics, and community mental health centers, efforts have been made to educate both patients and families about the illness. Families are counseled about how to handle the symptoms seen in patients, such as anger, withdrawal, delusions, hallucinations, and bizarre behavior. They also are educated about what to do in case of an emergency. It has been shown that the amount of "expressed emotion" in a family has a bearing on the recurrence and severity of schizophrenia. Counseling in the reduction of such emotional excesses among family members has been found to be of considerable value in reducing the outcome of schizophrenia.

Some patients attend a self-help group called Recovery, which can be helpful. It is a national organization run by former patients according to principles established by Dr. Abraham Low, as noted in his book *Mental Health Through Will Training*. Dr. Low contended that patients can become much more comfortable with their illness if they adopt his way of looking at symptoms. For example, a given symptom may be "distressing but not dangerous." He offers many aphorisms that patients can use when they are under stress.

In recent years, the families of patients who are seriously mentally ill have formed an influential group called the National Alliance for the Mentally Ill (NAMI). This group has as its mission the eradication of mental illness through research, for which it solicits funds. The group also is politically involved in advocating support for the mentally ill at the state and national levels. NAMI is a grass roots organization that is a strong force in helping those who have debilitating mental illnesses such as schizophrenia and bipolar disorder.

Research is being done on the causes of schizophrenia by the National Institute of Mental Health in Bethesda, Maryland, and by the major universities throughout the country. Researchers are pursuing genetic studies for the purpose of obtaining more accurate data for genetic counseling. Others are researching new drugs in an attempt to discover more effective drugs that have fewer side effects than those of earlier antipsychotic drugs. Some other researchers are focusing on the psychological and social reasons for the development of schizophrenia.

What Can Families, Friends, and Caregivers Do?

What can families, friends, and caregivers do for schizophrenic patients? First, I suggest that relatives, friends, and caregivers obtain as much information about schizophrenia as they can. Becoming educated about this mental illness is not difficult. There are numerous books on schizophrenia written for the general public. Another means of gaining information and insight into the illness is through groups such as NAMI. This group includes mentally ill patients and their families. There are local and state chapters of this organization. The purpose of NAMI is to disseminate information about mental illness, to lobby legislators, and to solicit money for research on serious mental disorders.

Asking questions of the treating psychiatrist also is helpful, but this should only be done with patients' full consent.

Participation in support groups for those caring for patients with schizophrenic disorders is important. Learning about this illness can make schizophrenia easier to handle on a day-to-day basis.

Caregivers can be helpful in making certain that patients take their medications at the correct times and in the right amounts. By themselves, patients often do not comply with instructions for medications.

When talking to patients, caregivers should learn to speak in short sentences, using simple concrete language. Long discussions do not hold the interest of patients who are acutely ill. Calmness is important, even when patients' behavior is out of the ordinary. Caregivers also should encourage patients to continue to socialize as much as possible.

Finally, patients themselves often know what is most helpful to them. Maintaining communication with the patients is useful, but patients also need their space and should not be badgered with constant "helping" by relatives, friends, and caregivers.

CHAPTER 16

OTHER PSYCHOTIC DISORDERS

In addition to schizophrenia and bipolar disorder, there are several other disorders that are seen in hospitals, clinics, and psychiatrists' offices. Patients with these other disorders have a psychosis that requires aggressive treatment.

The following disorders are included in the classification of schizophrenia and other psychotic disorders in DSM-IV. Also included are psychotic disorder due to a general medical condition, substance-induced psychotic disorder, and psychotic disorder not otherwise specified.

Schizophreniform Disorder

As the name implies, schizophreniform disorder is like schizophrenia. In the past, schizophreniform disorder was included in the American Psychiatric Association's classification for schizophrenia. Although the symptoms are similar, schizophreniform disorder is distinguished from schizophrenia by a shorter duration (less than 6 months from onset to resolution) and more acute symptoms. There may be only one episode, or several, of schizophreniform disorder in the lifetime of patients, but most patients are relatively free of symptoms between episodes. The treatment of the disorder is similar to that of schizophrenia.

Case Example

Jill came to see me about a stressful situation at her job. Many organizational changes at work were creating stress and anxiety for her. In the course of my inquiring into her background and medical history, she told me that at the age of 28 she had experienced a sudden onset of confusion, auditory hallucinations, and paranoid ideas about the people at work. She had been hospitalized for several weeks, treated with antipsychotic medication, and followed up for several months by a psychiatrist. Her psychiatrist's diagnosis at that time was schizophrenic reaction, acute (old terminology; this illness is now called schizophreniform disorder).

Since that time, she had married and had reared two children, and she was now employed as an office manager in a large firm. During the interval since her acute illness, she had never experienced any of the symptoms of psychosis.

After careful examination, I concluded that she showed no symptoms of her past illness. Her current situation was temporary and was a reaction to her job stress. After about 10 sessions of psychotherapy, during which she continued working, and a mild tranquilizer, she was free of symptoms and was functioning well again. She did not have schizophrenia.

It is important that schizophreniform disorder is distinguished from the more serious and chronic schizophrenia. In the past, patients like Jill were informed that they had schizophrenia, and they carried this label with them for a lifetime. Patients with schizophreniform disorder now can be told that they do not have schizophrenia, and although symptoms may return, if they are treated early, hospitalization and loss of work can be avoided or reduced to a minimum. On occasion, this illness can be prolonged and may deteriorate into schizophrenia.

Brief Psychotic Disorder

Brief psychotic disorder is caused by a sudden event that brings on symptoms of a psychosis. Traumas such as loss of a loved one, a major disaster, or a severe accident can precipitate the illness.

Although the disorder has a sudden onset, it is short in duration, usually lasting a few days to a month. Delusions, hallucinations, confusion, and disorganized thinking may be present. It is known to occur more often in persons with histrionic and borderline personality disorders, which are discussed in Chapter 12 in this volume.

Brief psychotic disorder is brought on mostly by emotional factors rather than by organic or biological influences.

Schizoaffective Disorder

There are some patients who do not have distinct forms of schizophrenia or bipolar disorder; rather, they may show symptoms of both. Hallucinations, delusions, and disorders in thinking are present along with disturbances in mood—either depression or mania. Generally, psychiatrists try to treat the predominant symptoms. The prognosis is poor and the illness tends to be chronic. Schizoaffective disorder is uncommon, and the diagnosis is not used much.

Delusional Disorder

The main symptoms of delusional disorder are paranoid ideas. They may involve the fear of being harmed or killed, the fear of impending disaster, the belief that others are plotting against the patients, or any other paranoid beliefs. These delusions also may involve pathological jealousy, grandiosity, or thoughts of being persecuted. Delusional disorder differs from schizophrenia because of the absence of symptoms such as hallucinations, disordered thinking, bizarre behavior, or inappropriate affect (feelings).

Patients with delusional disorder are hypersensitive, have low self-esteem, and have trouble trusting others. During paranoid states, patients become isolated and blame others for their problems.

In the past, one form of delusional disorder was called paranoia. In this illness, individuals have delusions about a particular subject (e.g., communism, germ warfare, different races) while functioning normally in most other respects. Delusional disorder is difficult to treat and may be present for years.

Shared Psychotic Disorder

Shared psychotic disorder (shared paranoid disorder), as the name implies, is diagnosed when an individual lives with a person who is paranoid and comes to believe in the same delusions. Shared psychotic disorder can occur among friends, relatives, or groups. It most often occurs with sisters living together. The first person has the primary illness and is dominant, and the other person or persons depend on him or her in various ways. An example of group behavior in which delusions were shared is the Jonestown catastrophe; many people committed suicide because of shared beliefs with a paranoid leader. A similar tragedy occurred among the Branch Davidians, a group led by a delusional leader. The deaths of the Davidians differed from the Jonestown deaths in that they were forced by the intrusion of government forces.

Treatment

The psychotic disorders are treated according to the patients' symptoms. Patients with any one of the psychotic disorders require antipsychotic medication and possibly a short stay in a hospital. The prescribed drugs are given to alleviate symptoms and control excessive behaviors while allowing patients to recover. The psychiatrist usually involves patients with psychotic disorders in supportive psychotherapy as well.

Schizoaffective, shared psychotic, and some delusional disorders usually become chronic and do not respond well to treatment. Schizophreniform disorder and brief psychotic disorder are generally of short duration and have a favorable prognosis.

What Can Families, Friends, and Caregivers Do?

When severe paranoid symptoms are present, caregivers often are not able to help a great deal, particularly if the caregivers are part of the patients' paranoid delusions. The best approach caregivers can take is to get the patients to a psychiatrist as soon as possible.

In general, the more acute the symptoms, the better the prognosis. During the acute phases of psychotic disorders, families, friends, and caregivers can give support to patients, who need to maintain their connections to those with whom they are close. It is most important that caregivers consult with the treating psychiatrist or other mental health professional regarding communication with patients. Support from others for patients in crisis cannot be overemphasized.

It also is helpful for caregivers to know something about the psychotic disorders because they differ widely in terms of prognosis. When caregivers are informed, they can make better judgments about their interactions with those for whom they are caring.

As with other severe illnesses, it is most important for the friends and family of those who have psychotic illnesses to support the psychiatrist's administration of medications and encourage the proper use of these drugs.

CHAPTER 17

DELIRIUM, DEMENTIA, AND AMNESTIC AND OTHER COGNITIVE DISORDERS

The disorders of the brain resulting from temporary or permanent injury used to be called organic brain disorders. This term is no longer used because of the implication that illnesses such as schizophrenia and others are not caused at all by biological problems. Recent research has shown that many of the disorders previously thought to be purely psychological have some biological basis.

The disorders are now broken down into the following four categories:

1. *Delirium.* Delirium is an alteration in consciousness and cognition that is usually short in duration. Visual hallucinations and confusion are often present.
2. *Dementia.* Dementia includes many cognitive deficiencies and memory problems. Confusion, disorientation, and recent memory loss are common.

3. *Amnestic disorder.* Memory loss, without other cognitive deficits, is the main feature of amnestic disorder. The disorder can occur from illnesses such as traumatic injury to the brain, stroke, and toxins.

4. *Other cognitive disorders.* Other cognitive disorders may be due to a general medical condition or substance-induced problems.

Case Example

Some years ago, I was supervising a psychiatric resident physician in an acute care hospital. He reported to me that a patient had been admitted the previous night in a psychotic state. She was confused, had paranoid delusions, was extremely overactive, and was difficult to control. She had symptoms not unlike those of many other patients whom we regularly saw on our unit. The resident noticed that her skin was dry, scaly, and thick, and her hair was sparse and coarse. She had a rapid pulse and her eyes appeared wide open and red. He said that her skin and hair reminded him of those of patients who had hypothyroidism. However, she showed none of the expected mental symptoms of hypothyroidism, such as slow movements, depression, and lack of energy. We ordered thyroid tests and when we received the results, the picture became clear. Her thyroid level was markedly elevated. We subsequently learned that she had been depressed and had taken a large overdose of Synthroid (levothyroxine), a thyroid medication. She had many of the mental and some physical symptoms of hyperthyroidism, although she did not have the disease as such. We treated her hyperactivity with tranquilizers and allowed the thyroid level to return to average levels, at which time she regained her healthy mental state.

Hypothyroidism and hyperthyroidism (in this case, due to an overdose of thyroid medication) are common organic diseases with mental symptoms. The patient had a complex organic illness that resembled a mental illness such as delusional disorder or schizophreniform disorder. However, the psychosis that occurred was due to toxic reaction to the drug Synthroid (levothyroxine).

Physicians often see patients with physical symptoms that are primarily due to emotional stress. It has been estimated that one-third of the complaints for which patients see physicians are stress related. Another one-third of patients have organic illnesses, such as stomach ulcers or asthma, that are affected by stress, whereas the remaining one-third have strictly organic illnesses. The latter group of illnesses, of course, can produce considerable stress too, but the stress is secondary to the illness—as with the psychological effects of having cancer. It is important for physicians to be aware of the true nature of an illness and to determine whether the origin of the malady is essentially organic or emotional.

Overview

It has long been recognized that many diseases of the brain are due to physical causes. Toxins, vitamin deficiencies, alcohol, and drugs are common causes of poor brain functioning. Basically, the brain chemistry is altered, but whatever the cause, it always involves either a temporary or permanent interference with brain function. Alcohol is an example of a substance that interferes with brain function. In small doses, alcohol usually has a pleasant but temporary effect on the person. The response is completely reversible. When alcohol is taken in excess, it has a far more dramatic effect on the mind, and the result may not be temporary if the alcohol is abused long enough. Chronic abuse leads to the destruction of nerve cells and permanent damage of the brain.

In Alzheimer's disease, certain abnormalities occur in the brain, and normal brain tissue is replaced. As tissue is replaced in the frontal lobes of the brain, patients with Alzheimer's disease lose their memory and have difficulty knowing the date and time and even the place where they reside. As the disease becomes worse, behavioral and cognitive changes occur. This dreaded illness affecting the older population comes on slowly and with little warning. The cause is not yet known, but researchers are moving closer to discovering what goes wrong in Alzheimer's disease.

In brain tumors, the abnormal tissue pushes against the normal brain tissue because of the confined space within the skull. Depending on which areas of the brain are affected, various symptoms follow. For example, if the tumor is in the back of the brain in the occipital area, disturbances in vision are likely to occur. If the tumor is in the motor area of the parietal lobe, the result would be difficulty with muscle coordination or spastic muscle movements. Some tumors can be treated in a variety of ways if they are accessible by surgery or treatable by X ray or chemotherapy.

Another common disease affecting the brain is arteriosclerosis. In this disease, circulation is compromised by a narrowing of the blood vessels in the brain. The result may be a blood clot, a thrombus, or bleeding from a large or small blood vessel. Depending on where in the brain the clot, thrombus, or bleeding occurs, certain brain cells will be affected. The corresponding brain functioning will be impaired, sometimes temporarily but often permanently. Although arteriosclerosis usually occurs in older persons, it can occur in young people when congenital blood vessel disease exists or in association with certain disorders such as diabetes.

A discussion of the many cognitive disorders is beyond the scope of this chapter. To show the range of diseases that affect the brain, I review the general causes of these disorders in the following discussions. There are many causes, but they can be summarized by the mnemonic *DEMENTIA.*

D reminds us of drug abuse. Drugs of abuse include a variety of illicit or street drugs that are used especially by young people in our society. Alcohol also must be mentioned because it is one of the most abused drugs in the world. Many people abuse over-the-counter drugs as well. In addition, drugs prescribed by physicians are frequently abused. Tranquilizers, sedatives, and medication for pain are among the most frequently abused. Recently, steroids have been used by athletes to build muscle mass for bodybuilding; these drugs are potentially harmful. Other drugs, such as cortisone derivatives, cardiac drugs, and thyroid drugs, can alter brain function and cause mental symptoms. Finally, drug interactions can be both physically and mentally harmful and must be carefully watched by the physician. These drug interactions are particularly common among older individuals.

E is for emotional disorders. There are many stress-related symptoms that can mimic organic disorders. For example, depression as a predominant symptom can be the result of hypothyroidism, Addison's disease, or a brain tumor. The psychiatrist must be certain that he or she has considered these possibilities before assuming that the illness is due to emotional conflicts. In older persons, depression can have the appearance of dementia, with confusion, recent memory loss, and poor functioning. Treating the basic depression can relieve completely the so-called pseudodementia.

Severe anxiety, especially in older individuals, can cause confusion, some loss of memory, and temporary disorientation. Even sudden changes, such as moving from home to a hospital, can cause a temporary confusion and disorientation in older patients. Many symptoms resulting from various stressors can appear to be organic, and organic diseases often may resemble emotional disorders.

M stands for endocrine or metabolic disorders. Hypothyroidism (underactive thyroid), hyperthyroidism (overactive thyroid), diabetes, hypoglycemia (low blood sugar), pituitary and parathyroid diseases, and adrenal tumors all can cause symptoms that affect the brain. They may first appear to be symptoms of anxiety or depression, or they may cause unusual thoughts or behaviors. Emotional changes may be quite marked. To differentiate these organic diseases from emotional illnesses and other mental disorders, the physician must rely on many laboratory tests to help find the origin of the problem. But even with our sophisticated diagnostic tools, errors in diagnosis can be made, particularly in the early stages of an illness. For example, a brain tumor in the frontal lobe of the brain can begin as depression with or without headaches. If a depressed patient were seen by a psychiatrist and the patient had no other symptoms, the physician might not suspect a tumor. From a practical point of view, it makes little sense to do expensive procedures on every patient who is depressed. However, if some physical symptoms such as severe headaches, nausea, vomiting, loss of balance, and dizziness are also present, a diagnostic study certainly would be indicated to rule out the possibility of a brain tumor.

Sometimes it takes a while for an illness to develop to the point of being clearly recognizable. Symptoms such as anxiety, depression, paranoid ideas, and behavioral changes often are seen in association with organic mental disorders.

E represents diseases of the eyes and ears. These sense organs permit us to constantly assess our environment. Without seeing and hearing what is happening, a person can develop emotional symptoms. For example, a hearing loss can cause an older person to develop paranoid ideas about his or her family or associates. Poor vision can be upsetting and in some cases can make a person suspicious. Loss of either of these special senses can lower an individual's self-esteem, particularly in an older individual.

N is for nutritional problems. Among young people, nutritional deficiencies may be hard to discover, even if their diets are far from ideal. Many adults consume too much caffeine in coffee and colas, possibly bringing on headaches and nervousness. Excessive sugar can sometimes cause hyperglycemia followed by a rebound hypoglycemia in those who are susceptible. But these are temporary disturbances. Because of improved nutrition, the more serious vitamin deficiencies such as pellagra, beriberi (vitamin B complex deficiency), and scurvy (vitamin C deficiency) are not often seen in those who live in developed countries. Deficiencies of these important vitamins can cause organic brain disorders.

Poor nutrition can be found among older persons, alcohol and drug abusers, the homeless, and patients with certain medical conditions such as severe diarrhea. A variety of organic symptoms, ranging from short-term memory loss, poor coordination, and inability to think clearly to loss of consciousness, can occur. If individuals with poor nutrition come to medical caregivers, the deficiencies can be detected easily, and the necessary vitamin and mineral supplements can be supplied.

T reminds us of trauma and tumors. Although head trauma can occur at any age, it is especially common among the older population. Head trauma also is likely to be seen among alcoholic persons and those who abuse drugs. The symptoms that occur from head trauma are varied depending on the degree and location of the injury. Head traumas can cause temporary or permanent malfunction of the brain.

Brain tumors cause symptoms because they press on normal nerve tissue and prevent areas of the brain from functioning. Sometimes, tumors may be present without many symptoms. For example, a slow-growing tumor, such as a meningioma, in the frontal lobe of the brain just behind a person's eye might cause no symptoms other than depression. Such a benign tumor could be present for several years and not be detected. When other symptoms such as headaches and vomiting occur, a psychiatrist would suspect the presence of a tumor and would order the necessary tests to determine whether the patient has a tumor.

Tumors can be slow growing and benign or rapidly growing and malignant. The latter type can come on suddenly, within weeks, and result in death within months. New techniques have been developed to diagnose these tumors. These are described in detail later in this chapter.

I represents infection. Diseases such as brain abscesses, meningitis, or encephalitis may be caused by bacteria, viruses, or other forms of infection. Infections can come from the environment or from another organ in the body, such as the heart. When the heart is inflamed with endocarditis, small bits of infected material in the form of emboli may go to the brain and cause infection there. The brain also can be affected by the presence of disease in other organs such as the lungs. When this occurs, as in emphysema, the supply of oxygen to the brain may be insufficient, resulting in symptoms of disorientation, confusion, and poor memory.

Finally, *A* stands for arteriosclerosis. In this condition, the flow of blood through the arteries is compromised because the vessels are narrowed or have clots in them. As a result, there is not enough blood flow to the brain. In this malnourished state, the brain is deprived of oxygen, and memory loss occurs along with confusion and disorientation. If this condition is prolonged, eventually personality deterioration occurs.

How Brain Disorders Are Diagnosed

The physician who suspects a brain disorder must first obtain from the patient a history of the onset of the illness. This information can give valuable clues as to the presence of a serious brain disorder. Next, certain laboratory tests would be needed to rule out many diseases, such as drug or alcohol abuse, trauma, nutritional deficiencies, or endocrine diseases. The tests usually can help the physician to rule out or suspect these diseases and can help in the diagnosis. Obtaining spinal fluid for testing is valuable. Determining spinal fluid pressure, the chemical contents of the fluid, and the presence of infection in the fluid is important for establishing diagnoses.

The recent invention of new radiological techniques has done more than anything else to help in diagnosing brain abnormalities. Traditional X rays of the skull are of limited value because such procedures only show bone abnormalities. When I first became a physician, a technique called pneumoencephalography was being used. In this procedure, air was injected into the spinal column, where it was allowed to displace some of the spinal fluid. This air could be detected on the X ray. If tumors or abscesses were displacing areas that normally were filled with fluid, this would show up as an abnormality on the X-ray films. But this method was of limited value in making accurate diagnoses.

The next tool invented was the brain scan. Although it had its limitations, it was another step toward assisting diagnosis. The physician injected a radioactive material into a vein, and shortly after, X rays of the brain were taken and the blood vessels of the brain were highlighted. Any abnormality in the vessels, as well as a deformity of a vessel representing something pushing on the artery or vein, would be viewed as possible disease.

Later, computed tomography (CT) was invented. Using X-ray techniques and computer technology, a physician could see an image of the soft tissues of the brain at any level. Comparing normal and abnormal brain pictures, the radiologist was able to make comparisons and diagnose brain pathology or its absence.

The next step in refining diagnosis of brain disorders was nuclear magnetic resonance scanning or magnetic resonance imaging (MRI). In MRI, a radio signal is sent to the brain in a uniform magnetic field. When the polarity of the magnetic field is momentarily changed, the brain can be seen from various planes and directions via a computer monitor. As a result, many forms of brain pathology can now be diagnosed. For example, the lining of nerve tracts can now be viewed, and diseases such as multiple sclerosis, in which segments of the covering of nerve fibers are missing, can be detected. It was not possible to diagnose such conditions with previous radiological techniques. Thus, great gains have been made toward earlier diagnosis and treatment. The sooner a diagnosis can be made, the more rapidly a possible treatment can be determined.

In this country, CT scans and MRI are available at major health centers and at many community hospitals.

The latest innovation in radiological techniques is the positron emission tomography (PET) scan. It is used for research at this time and is not available for use in clinical medicine. The PET scan has a different function from that of either the CT or MRI scan. CT and MRI measure and show the structure, form, and size of organs of the body, including the brain. The PET scan, however, measures brain function. It can determine what areas of the brain are active and to what degree. With the PET scan, researchers can study the metabolism of the brain. Glucose is labeled with a positron-emitting isotope, such as fluorine 19, and it is injected into a vein of the person to be studied. The PET scanner is then able to view the brain along various axes. The observer can tell what area of the brain is using the injected glucose; it shows on the screen in the form of various colors. The amount of glucose consumed can be measured, and the site of action can be located. For example, if the person's eyes are closed, it shows little activity in the occipital area. When the eyes are open, bright colors show in the occipital region, thus indicating that this area is active. Similar studies can be done on the brain to study the metabolism of other substances such as drugs or amino acids. As a result of such research, a great deal of information about the metabolism of the brain and its various functions is being determined. Such information will be useful in the future for the diagnosis and treatment of organic brain disease.

A simpler diagnostic tool related to the PET scan is single photon emission computed tomography (SPECT). It is used in certain settings for diagnostic studies. In time, SPECT may be used more generally.

Cognitive Disorders Appearing As Emotional Disorders

When counseling patients with emotional problems, the psychotherapist must always be aware of the possibility of organic illness lurking in the background. It is interesting that some of the most severe forms of mental illness such as schizophrenia may have few physical components. In contrast, many patients with severe physical disease such as cancer may have relatively few mental or emotional symptoms. In most illnesses that therapists treat, there are combined organic and psychological factors. The important part of the puzzle is to ferret out the basic reason for the illness.

In the following case examples, I illustrate how what initially appeared to be an emotional disorder later was diagnosed as an organic disease.

Case Example 1

A 40-year-old man, Jeff, came into my office with his wife to talk about his depression. His symptoms began about 5 weeks before this visit and were getting worse. He also was becoming somewhat paranoid about his boss and other people at work. Jeff had had an episode of depression several years ago. It had been treated by a psychiatrist, and he had recovered in about 6 weeks. His current illness appeared to be similar to the first depression.

I chose to treat Jeff with weekly psychotherapy and some medication. Ordinarily, I would have expected some improvement in 4–5 weeks of treatment. However, Jeff's symptoms only became worse. I decided to place him in a local hospital for further evaluation. I had an internist examine him and order a series of tests. The results of one of the screening tests were reported as abnormal. Meanwhile, Jeff's condition was growing worse. He developed many organic symptoms, including memory deficits, disorientation, and confusion. All of his symptoms suggested MRI of the brain was necessary. The result was surprising. It revealed vasculitis, an inflammation of the blood vessels of the brain. Vasculitis is a serious illness, the origin of which is unknown. The diagnosis was confirmed by another consultant and treatment was begun. After some initial improvement, Jeff was sent home. However, he never recovered completely and had to depend on continued monitoring for treatment of his organic illness. What appeared to be a typical depression with some paranoid ideas turned out to be a serious life-threatening physical illness.

Case Example 2

A 72-year-old man, Harold, was referred to me by his family physician. Harold had lost his wife 2 years ago. He had a good deal of support from his seven children, all of whom lived close to his home. But despite all of the encouragement from friends and family, Harold still seemed to be grieving his deceased wife. He was depressed and anxious, and he tended to stay by himself most of the time.

With the symptoms that were present, it seemed like a good idea to place Harold on an antidepressant to help lift his mood, while I investigated his prolonged grief. After about 6 months, Harold appeared to be much improved. He seemed to have overcome his grief, and he was socializing more and was no longer depressed. I began to see him less frequently and assumed that he was well on the way to recovery.

Then, one day Harold came in looking a bit different. I could not put my finger on the quality of the change. I asked him how he had felt in the last 2 weeks. He replied, "This week I took a foot stepwards." I did not regard this as an ordinary mistake such as "I took a step forward" although meaning "backward." Rather, he was confusing two words and misplacing them in the sentence. I listened further and heard only a trace of misspoken words in that session. Thereafter, I occasionally heard other grossly abnormal misstatements. It made me suspect an organic illness. I asked him to go to a neurologist, who at the time ordered a CT scan. It did not show any abnormality. The neurologist reported no organic disease on his examination, but Harold's problems with speech continued to grow worse, as I observed at our infrequent visits. One year later, the neurologist reexamined Harold and concluded that he had early Alzheimer's disease.

Harold's initial illness was undoubtedly an emotional disorder that responded to traditional treatment, but simultaneously he was beginning to develop an organic syndrome, which at the beginning was only manifested by a speech disorder. It is not uncommon to see two illnesses in the same patient, one an emotional or mental illness and the other an organic illness.

What Can Families, Friends, and Caregivers Do?

First, it is important for anyone in contact with persons who have organic and/or emotional disorders to be aware that for their mental and emotional lives to operate well, an intact brain is required. This statement may seem self-evident, but frequently, caregivers do not recognize subtle symptoms that indicate brain pathology. It is tempting to see individuals' emotional outbursts or unusual thinking as the result of job or family pressures or any other stressors that may consume the individuals. But behavior is always the result of a combination of the stresses imposed. The closer caregivers are to the individuals, the more likely they are to blame emotional stresses for alterations in behavior and ignore the possibility of other causes.

In general, organic illnesses bring out the best and the worst in people. Persons who are emotionally dependent become more dependent. Those with an irritable strain become more irritable. Easygoing, relaxed, and laid-back individuals will usually be true to these traits when ill, whereas angry, disgruntled persons will become more so. These traits also are maintained during the aging process. The positive and negative traits that are recognized in the middle-aged adult will become exaggerated as the person ages. In senile patients, the pattern of behavior becomes even more pronounced. Caregivers should be aware that organic illnesses bring out the best and worst in their patients so that there are no surprises as they maintain involvement with patients.

As patients lose physical or mental abilities, they may react differently to the same loss. For example, when an athletic man or woman suddenly loses the ability to perform his or her favorite activity, it has far more meaning than when a person who has no interests in athletics loses that same ability. Similarly, if an accountant has a mild stroke and loses some of his or her mathematical ability, it is of immense importance. If a laborer had a stroke and lost mathematical ability, it would have less significance.

Caregivers must be aware of a patient's specific loss. They must appreciate how a particular loss affects that individual and interpret the loss in terms of his or her particular interests and concerns. Sometimes, caregivers project themselves into the situation and react as though the loss were easy to endure because the caregivers think that it would be easy for them to manage.

Illness often brings on exaggerated dependency. Caregivers should be aware of this fact and not permit patients to become too dependent. Patients should be encouraged to be as self-sufficient as their illness allows. In the acute phases of illness, less can be expected. When improvement occurs, patients can do more. The caregivers' goals should be to view each patient individually and try to deal with the changing emotions and alterations in physical abilities as treatment continues.

Caring for aged parents is one of the hardest tasks for adult children. At first the job is not complicated. Mom and Dad become increasingly dependent on the children, and their needs are easily met. With increasing age, a parent may become forgetful, confused, and disoriented. Now the trouble begins. At these times, many adult children have difficulty taking charge. Why? It is hard to stop the old pattern of reacting like a child—even to the aged parent. We all naturally behave as we have done for many years. If Mom or Dad demands something strongly enough, the tendency is to give in for the sake of "peace" and grant the wish, regardless of how unreasonable it may be.

One of the first of these demands is the issue of driving. For example, if an 85-year-old man has memory deficits and is at times confused, he obviously should not be driving. But I have seen adult children have difficulty denying a father's request to "just drive around the neighborhood." In these situations, it is important for the adult child to realize that the parent no longer has good judgment and is making an unreasonable and perhaps dangerous request. There comes a time when the son or daughter must take on the parental role and become firm in directing the parent's behavior. In essence, when the parent is acting like a child, he or she must be handled and directed firmly as one would handle a child.

If Mom is using a knife improperly in the kitchen and is in danger of cutting herself, the knife should be taken away, even if she objects. Mom can do other tasks that are not potentially harmful. Or if Dad is confused and in a moment of poor judgment thinks he can clean out the gutters on a two-story house as he has done for years, he should be prevented from doing so. The ladder should be removed and another job given. It is a time to be firm, to take charge, and to assume the parental role. When the adult child reaches this level of caregiving and in effect becomes the parent, life becomes much simpler and the emotional impact less difficult to handle. I have seen many families go through this transition successfully. It takes a bit of thought, determination, and practice, but it can be done.

PART IV

TREATMENT OF EMOTIONAL AND MENTAL ILLNESSES

CHAPTER 18

HOW A PSYCHIATRIST HELPS

There are many kinds of counselors in the mental health field: social workers, psychologists, psychiatric nurse practitioners, pastoral counselors, activity therapists, drug and alcohol counselors, rehabilitation and vocational counselors, and many others. Since I am a psychiatrist, in this chapter I focus on what I know best—what a psychiatrist does.

The Psychiatrist's Background

After 4 years of college and 4 more years of medical school, the physician interested in psychiatry must take 4 years of psychiatric residency training in hospitals and clinics.

The training begins with hospital care of severely ill patients, who have illnesses such as schizophrenia, manic-depressive (bipolar) disorder, panic disorder, various psychosomatic disorders, alcohol and drug abuse, and neurological problems. These disorders are diagnosed and treated under the supervision of senior staff psychiatrists.

Many hours of psychotherapy are also conducted on an outpatient basis with patients who have neurotic problems, personality disorders, adjustment disorders, and other problems. The patients with more severe illnesses also may be treated in outpatient settings. These patients are seen in weekly psychotherapy sessions or less often, depending on their particular disorder. Many hours of clinical supervision are included in the resident's work.

In academic lectures, resident psychiatrists receive instruction in the diagnosis of various child and adult psychiatric disorders. Treatment of patients in individual, group, and family therapies includes psychotherapy and psychotropic medications.

Psychiatrists learn and practice the various forms of psychotherapy, including supportive, behavioral, cognitive, and dynamic or psychoanalytically oriented psychotherapy. (These therapies are discussed in Chapter 19 in this volume.) Although there are other therapies that are used in the psychotherapist's world, the foregoing therapies are the main types in use at this time. Most residency training in psychiatry is eclectic. Trainees are exposed to and use the available therapies so that they do not use one form of psychotherapy exclusively. I believe that no one method of treatment is applicable to all patients. People are too complicated to be placed into one treatment modality. Everyone does not respond to the same kind of psychotherapy. For example, relatively few people can benefit from a lengthy psychoanalysis although it is helpful when properly used. Others benefit greatly from one form of short-term therapy or another. Still others need to deal with unconscious forces and require a more dynamic type of psychotherapy. The form of treatment should be appropriate for the diagnosis, as well as the practical issues of time and financial concerns.

Other topics included in the training of psychiatrists are ethics, forensic psychiatry, the interplay between neurological and psychiatric problems, and the effect of cultural experiences on mental health or illness. After completing the required 4 years of residency training and practicing for several years, most psychiatrists take an examination to qualify as board certified by the American Board of Psychiatry and Neurology. Board certification is not a requirement for practicing psychiatry, but most psychiatrists do take the examination. In addition, many psychiatrists undergo a formal psychoanalysis with a senior psychoanalyst to work out any problems they may have in their own emotional life, as well as to assist them in their work with patients. Psychoanalysis of psychiatrists is not a requirement for their practicing psychiatry, but it is recommended to round out psychiatric training.

Basic Theoretical Assumptions

In the following discussions, I describe several basic theories of the mind on which dynamic (psychoanalytically oriented) psychotherapy is based. I include the theory of the unconscious, psychic determinism, resistance, transference, countertransference, and defense mechanisms.

Theory of the Unconscious

Most psychiatrists and psychotherapists, other than those who practice behavioral and cognitive therapy exclusively, accept the presence of the unconscious as a significant force in the emotional life of humans. Freud was the first to apply this theory to the specific treatment of mental disorders. However, it was not a new phenomenon in terms of the experience of humankind. Literature, mythology, and religious writings all feature the forces of good and evil in humans and among the gods. Saint Paul, speaking of these warring factions within himself, as recorded in the King James Version of the Bible, said: "For the good that I would I do not: but the evil which I would not, that I do." That is, the conscious mind wills to do certain things, but the deep unconscious forces often have their way in our behavior.

Freud said that the unconscious is manifested in many ways—in dreams (the "royal road to the unconscious"), in common errors that we make in our speech and behavior, in how we repeat behaviors that have existed in the past (repetition-compulsion), and in the inconsistencies in our daily living. The unconscious is dramatically illustrated in the stories *The Strange Case of Dr. Jekyll and Mr. Hyde* and *The Three Faces of Eve*. These are stories of characters who have exceptional behaviors, but they provide good examples of the conflicts causing contrasting behaviors within the characters.

Psychic Determinism

In his classic work on psychic determinism, "The Psychopathology of Everyday Life," Freud gave many examples from daily experience as to how the unconscious operates. The basic theory is that nothing happens in our mental life without some prior cause or combination of causes, even if we are not immediately able to ascertain what they might be. No thought or act is totally spontaneous. Even in various acts of creativity, there are mental or emotional antecedents. All of our acts are based on some past experience. From his clinical work in hypnosis, Freud postulated that the symptoms that a patient has are the result of mental conflicts between the superego (conscience) and the id impulses of sex and aggression. He invented the treatment called psychoanalysis to ferret out the conscious and unconscious roots of the conflict.

The psychotherapy done by most psychotherapists is based on Freud's view of mental conflicts. Therefore, it is the job of the psychotherapist to figure out what causes the patient's neurotic behavior based on his or her conscious recall, as well as on his or her dreams and free association (i.e., whatever thoughts occur when the mind is allowed to wander in the process of therapy). Having discovered the patient's conflicts, the psychiatrist then proceeds to help the patient find alternative ways of dealing with his or her impulses, consistent with the patient's superego needs and cultural and environmental concerns.

Resistance

Resistance to the work of therapy is a common phenomenon. Although patients consciously want to improve and be free of conflicts and symptoms, often the changes are difficult. The old patterns persist, and there is a natural resistance to change. A preference for the known, the status quo, and the familiar is strongly felt in those who consciously want to improve their lives and feel better. In therapy, there is a constant tension between the mental desire to change and the unconscious holding on to past behaviors and feelings. This holding on is especially true of feelings. It is easier to alter a behavior than to change a feeling. When behaviors and feelings change for some time, a significant move has been made in the therapeutic process. A good therapist must present the reality of the patient's problem to him or her and must be an emotional catalyst to help the patient overcome conflicts through the course of the therapy.

Transference

In his analytic method, Freud discovered that feelings developed between him and the patients that he could not account for based on the reality of the therapeutic situation. Because of the intense nature of the analytic process, he found that patients had emotional reactions to him that were incongruous to what he expected. A young female patient expressed feelings of love; another expressed unprovoked anger. Others showed feelings that were not appropriate based on what was happening in the therapeutic hour. As a result of these observations, Freud developed the idea that patients were taking feelings and attitudes from the past and unconsciously *transferring* them into the present setting of therapy. For example, the intense erotic feelings of a female patient for her father years ago were unconsciously placed on the therapist. He later called this the *transference neurosis* and felt that it was a necessary part of the analytic process. Freud came to believe that the successful resolution of this transference was necessary for a cure to take place. Transference was a kind of reliving of the experience with the significant person in the past in which feelings were evoked with the therapist in the therapeutic setting and finally resolved in a conscious manner. In effect, it made the patients' unconscious erotic or aggressive feelings conscious. Through transference, patients could deal with their feelings more maturely instead of inappropriately. Dealing with feelings inappropriately resulted from repressed (unconsciously forgotten) childhood fantasies.

The following case example may be helpful in understanding this interesting phenomenon known as transference.

Case Example

Alice, age 40 years, came to seek help for her feelings of anxiety and depression. These symptoms were not overwhelming in the sense that she could not function at all. She was a schoolteacher and was managing to do her job adequately. But she continually felt that she could do better, if only she did not suffer from constant symptoms. In addition, she complained about her marriage, which she described as okay sometimes but only "so-so" most of the time. Whatever she had expected of marriage had not happened, although she could not put her finger on the exact problem.

Alice seemed to develop an initial positive relationship with me, although I felt that she was holding back—not revealing information to me and not expressing her feelings adequately. I asked her about this. To my surprise, she became angry, as though I were criticizing her severely. It was obvious that I had hit upon a sensitive area. She accused me of being like other men—always wanting to know everything and then telling nothing about themselves. In part, her statement was true because I had not told her anything significant about me, as is common in therapeutic situations. (In this sense, therapy is one-sided and not at all like a friendship in which feelings and attitudes are mutually shared.)

Gradually, Alice did reveal her feelings about the way men treated her. For some reason, about which she was very unclear, she believed men always took advantage of her. She always seemed to be expressing her feelings about men without their reciprocating. She was always doing things for them without a similar response from them. All of this made her angry and tense. As time went on and Alice reflected on this theme, she became aware that she had similar reactions to her husband and her supervisor, the school principal. Those men with whom she had only a casual relationship did not affect her this way. Only the men who were important in her life had this effect. In time, she realized that her father, and to some extent her mother, seemed to take advantage of her good nature. She had feelings of resentment toward them as well.

Given these underlying emotional reactions to the people in her life, it was not surprising that Alice had symptoms. The goal in therapy was to have Alice become aware of what she was doing to cause these repetitious feelings. Did she expect too much from people? Did she do too much for them and then feel disappointment when they did not respond in kind? Was she a patsy? Did people walk all over her only to have her resent them and be unable to confront them effectively? What could she realistically expect from those close to her? These were some of the questions that I asked Alice in our sessions.

As time went on, the picture became clear. Alice did overextend herself too many times to get into the good graces of others and have them like her. Eventually, she learned how to avoid this behavior and found out that people respected and liked her as much as before. As a result, Alice did not have to work as hard at her relationships with people, and she did not have the resentment toward them that she had previously felt. Although there were other problems of less importance, when Alice worked out the main issue, she felt relieved and her symptoms decreased and finally went away. On occasion, Alice had a resurgence of the symptoms, but the symptoms occurred only at times when she temporarily regressed to her former pattern of behavior.

Transference has come to be a valuable tool for the psychotherapist. It explains to the therapist the many overreactions of the patient. If the transference is positive, it can be a powerful force in permitting the patient to explore his or her conflicts and arrive at solutions for his or her life, as Alice did. Whatever happens in the transference usually has happened at some point in the patient's past.

When the transference is negative and the patient allows the exploration of these negative feelings, the therapist can determine why the patient becomes so inappropriately angry in circumstances that do not call for such a response. When the transference is positive and the patient becomes too emotionally involved with the therapist, the therapist can explore the feelings and relate them to similar emotional reactions to significant others in the patient's past. Thus, transference becomes one of the main forces at work toward healing the emotional wounds of the person's past.

Countertransference

Countertransference is the process by which the therapist unconsciously allows his or her feelings and attitudes from the past to come into the therapeutic situation. As a result of counter-transference, the therapist may overreact by becoming emotionally involved either negatively or positively with the patient. He or she may show signs of being too attached erotically to the patient, too overprotective, too dependent on the patient's return for sessions, or too attached in any other inappropriate manner. In a negative countertransference, the therapist becomes overly sensitive, angry, or sarcastic or in some other way displays that he or she is not maintaining the therapeutic relationship.

The following case example clarifies how countertransference works.

Case Example

One of my patients, Gary, had been in therapy for some time. I had helped him with symptoms of depression, but he continued to be overly dependent on me. I pointed this out to him and he tacitly acknowledged that this was so. However, it did not change his behavior. He continually complained about his job and his loneliness, and despite anything I could offer him in our sessions, he resisted moving ahead. He made no effort to change his behavior at work, nor did he do anything to get into contact with people so as to alleviate his loneliness. After months of his complaining that he was not feeling any better and his making no attempt at change, I became annoyed at him. I noticed that at the beginning of each session, I felt fine, but toward the end of the time with Gary, I felt angry and frustrated. At times I let Gary know that I felt this way; it had no effect on him.

Upon reflection, it became clear to me that my own feelings were getting in the way of therapy and that I was not doing Gary any favor by continuing to see him. When a patient comes to me for assistance, I should be able to help the patient and meet his or her needs. After a certain amount of time, the patient ought to feel better, and my need to help ought to be satisfied. In my work with Gary, he was getting nowhere, and I was feeling ineffective. (No one likes to feel this way at his or her job.) But my frustration was constant and an overreaction to the situation. I have been in somewhat similar situations before and have not reacted this way. I knew the problem was mine; I made the decision to ask the patient to see another therapist. Gary's reaction to this suggestion was that I was rejecting him. I explained that I understood how he felt, but that it would be in his own best interest to try to work with another therapist. He reluctantly did so.

After about 6 months in treatment with the new therapist, Gary was on his way toward recovery. He made some significant moves at work in the way in which he handled his boss and fellow employees, and as a result, he felt much better about himself. Gradually, he befriended others and developed a somewhat better social life. Within the year, Gary was no longer in need of therapy.

What was my problem with Gary? I am not entirely certain. It had something to do with his apparent helplessness in contrast to his own past ability to perform rather well. If he had had a lifelong dependence on others, I do not think I would have reacted to him in the same manner, but his inability to change emotionally at this stage of life seemed not to fit his potential to do so. I suspect that he touched on my own partially unconscious resistance to change, which is something I do not always want to face. Having recognized this negative countertransference, I thought it best that Gary work with another therapist.

It is important that psychotherapists have some knowledge of their own inner emotional life. After all, in sessions with patients, therapists have only their own personality and accumulated expertise with which to work. If a psychotherapist has only a limited awareness of his or her own personality deficits, therapeutic work with patients, who have their own emotional and mental hang-ups, can be difficult. For this reason, it is important for psychotherapists to have an analytic experience in which they spend some time being the patients. By doing so, they actually experience and live through these challenging transference and countertransference issues, thus making themselves more proficient in their work. Although personal psychoanalysis for every psychotherapist may not be practical, there are other therapeutic modalities that could give therapists the experience of being patients. These other modalities include cognitive and behavioral therapy, as well as group therapy.

Defense Mechanisms

In Chapter 7, I referred to Freud's concept of the neurosis in which he described the mental conflict that occurs between the id and the superego. In normal situations, people are able to repress the conflict enough so that no symptoms occur. Freud spoke of repression as one of the main defenses that individuals employ to avoid anxiety, but there are many others. In the following discussions, I review some of these common defense mechanisms, without providing an extensive list of defenses.

All defense mechanisms operate outside of our awareness; that is, our minds employ these defenses without our being aware of it (unconsciously). Some common defense mechanisms that we all use in our daily lives follow.

Repression. Repression is the mind's ability to forget or push back conflicts or problems that are facing the individual. It is, in effect, unconscious forgetting. The best example of repression is the following scenario, which I am certain you have experienced: You are terribly distraught about a current crisis in your life. You seem to be unable to forget about it. Suddenly, you realize that for the last 15 minutes you have not thought about the crisis at all. The awareness of the crisis was repressed for that brief time. Later, you notice that this repression occurs repeatedly. Without any conscious attempt on your part, your mind has been able to push away the crisis in order to permit you to carry on with the routine tasks that need to be done. The ability of your mind to repress conflicts and attend to urgent matters appears to be necessary for you to function.

Sublimation. Sublimation is the substitution of activities for the satisfaction of more primitive id (instinctual) impulses. For example, sexual and aggressive drives may be partially satisfied or delayed by the participation in sports or physical training.

Rationalization. Rationalization is the act of offering a socially acceptable reason for a given activity instead of stating the real or more basic reason for such behavior. For example, when adolescents say

"Everybody's doing it," they are stating a common shared belief, although untrue, for taking drugs or engaging in other behaviors of which adults may disapprove. By rationalizing, they justify their behaviors.

Intellectualization.   Intellectualization is the substitution of an idea or argument for an emotion. For example, when I once asked a patient how he felt about the fact that his best friend had died, he said that the chances of his friend living, given the disease he had, were statistically not good. Instead of telling me how he felt about the loss of his friend, he intellectualized the experience and gave a textbook response.

Some less common and more primitive defenses that the mind uses to maintain the integrity of the self (ego) follow.

Regression.   Regression may be seen in serious illnesses such as schizophrenia; the patient's behavior deteriorates and the patient regresses to a previous level of functioning. Childish or even infantile behavior can be seen, such as thumb sucking, soiling, or assuming the fetal position. Of course, we all experience lesser forms of regression, such as when we "play" during recreation or on vacation.

Projection.   Projection is placing blame onto another person for something that is emotionally a problem to the self. For example, a man may feel unconscious guilt about sexual thoughts or impulses regarding other women while accusing his wife of infidelity.

Denial.   Denial is the failure to admit that a serious problem exists. It may be seen in alcoholic patients, who, despite all the evidence that they are in serious trouble with drinking, nevertheless deny that they have a problem. Another example of this defense is seen in heavy smokers, who deny the health issues of their habit. In patients who have psychological problems, the observer can see destructive behaviors in which the patients engage, whereas the patients are not able to grasp the nature of their obvious deleterious conduct. Denial also is a common defense mechanism in couples with marriage problems.

Acting out.   In general, acting out refers to the attempt to re-solve an emotional problem from one arena of life by playing it out in another arena. For example, a marriage that is not meeting the emotional needs of an individual might prompt that person to have an affair. That is, instead of attempting to work out the prob-lem in the marriage, there is a substitute behavior in another place with another person. The problem is acted out rather than solved within the original setting. Another example is anger felt at the workplace, which often is carried home and displaced or acted out on the family.

There are other defense mechanisms that help explain the actions of people both in sickness and in health. (For further information on de-fense mechanisms, see the psychiatry textbooks listed in the Sug-gested Readings for this chapter at the end of this book.)

During the treatment process, psychiatrists need to be aware of the defenses used by their patients so that they may help their pa-tients get well. For example, the denial so commonly seen in alco-holic patients must be confronted directly by the psychiatrist. Going along with alcoholic patients' rationalizations about their illness and their denial of its very existence will only delay treatment. Failing to deal with the denial only serves to enable patients to go on drinking. As another example, if depressed patients constantly repress their anger, they may not be able to free themselves of their depression. They have to learn how to express their anger when that is the appro-priate emotion for a given situation.

Psychiatrists and other psychotherapists usually recognize the phenomena mentioned previously (i.e., the existence of the uncon-scious mind, psychic determinism, resistance, transference, coun-tertransference, and defense mechanisms). Therapists who use only behavioral or cognitive therapy do not use these concepts in their work with patients. However, it is difficult for these therapists to es-cape the use of these terms on occasion because these concepts have become so basic to psychiatric theory and practice.

Medications in the Treatment of Emotional and Mental Illnesses

The psychiatrist has another helpful tool to use in the treatment of emotionally and mentally ill patients: psychotropic drugs. Such medications have been found useful in treating patients who have psychoses, serious mood disorders, and various neuroses. The following discussion is an overview of the psychotropic medications used in psychiatry.

As background to the discussion and understanding of medications used in the mental health field, it is necessary to consider a few somewhat simplistic facts about brain anatomy and function. Researchers have only begun to scratch the surface in understanding how the brain works and how medications affect the brain on a cellular level and in terms of overall functioning. Although there have been many attempts to find cellular pathology in the more serious mental illnesses, there has been relatively little success. Minor changes have been found in the frontal lobes and elsewhere in the brains of schizophrenic patients. It is quite likely that there will be more findings regarding brain pathology in seriously mentally ill patients, but the bulk of the research is being done on the biochemical level within the basic cell structure of the brain.

The brain has several basic structures. The first is the neuron (nerve cell). Each neuron contains a cell body, which has a nerve fiber (axon) extending *away* from the cell, carrying nerve impulses out toward muscles, organs, or other parts of the brain. Another nerve fiber (dendrite) receives nerve impulses going *toward* the neuron. Dendrites have tiny branches that extend out to other brain structures.

All neurons have connections with other neurons by a space that is called a synapse. This space contains chemicals that transmit messages from one neuron to another. These chemicals are called neurotransmitters. The brain manufactures substances that synthesize these neurotransmitters, whereas other substances break them down, resulting in a continual renewal of these chemicals. In addition, other elements play a part in the synapse. Magnesium, sodium, calcium, and vitamins are among the substances that are important to metabolism in the brain.

Although there are a number of neurotransmitters, there are three that are especially important in the biochemistry of mental illness. They are serotonin, norepinephrine, and dopamine. Although the pathology of mental illnesses is far more complicated than we presently know, we are aware of some facts. In the mood disorders, serotonin and norepinephrine are lowered at the level of the synapses when serious depression is present. In contrast, these neurotransmitters are elevated in the manic phase of bipolar disorder. In order to treat these disorders, medications are given that affect the levels of these neurotransmitters. Therefore, antidepressants raise and antimanic drugs lower the levels of serotonin and norepinephrine. As these medications are given, there eventually is a corresponding improvement in patients. In addition, in patients who have acute schizophrenia, there is an excess of dopamine in the synapses of the brain. When the appropriate antipsychotic medications are given, these dopamine levels return to more normal levels. When this occurs, the symptoms of acute schizophrenia subside or may even disappear completely.

Although there may not be much evident cellular pathology in mental illnesses in comparison with other diseases, there appears to be a considerable biochemical disorder. This disorder can be corrected at least in part by the proper use of medications. With each passing year, researchers are discovering more about the complex mechanisms of the brain. As time goes on, the treatment of mental illnesses will be further refined and the clinical improvement in these illnesses will be marked.

It has been about 40 years since the first psychotropic medication was used. In the years before the 1950s, the psychiatrist had little choice in medications for the mentally ill. Various drugs were used by physicians and laypersons alike. Alcohol, nicotine, and caffeine were well known to affect mood, as were ether and morphine. Barbiturates were used liberally for sedation and sleep disorders. Sometimes they were also helpful in controlling the excesses of behavior among the mentally ill. But none of these drugs has any profound effect on the gross disturbances of mental illness.

In recent years, the use of psychotropic drugs for the mentally ill has had a tremendous effect on the ability of patients to recover from their illnesses sooner; many have remained well and are functioning better. Whether patients have disorders of mood, thinking, or behavior, psychotropic medications have profoundly changed the course of treatment for them. Many patients who formerly had to remain in psychiatric hospitals are now living at home or in shared homes for the mentally ill.

In general, there are four main types of drugs that are used for the emotionally and mentally ill. They are as follows:

1. *Antianxiety drugs.* Antianxiety drugs are used for the temporary relief of anxiety, panic, and phobic disorders. On occasion, these medications can be effective in preventing these conditions. Especially noteworthy is Xanax (alprazolam), used in preventing panic attacks. Other drugs in this category are Valium (diazepam), Librium (chlordiazepoxide), Ativan (lorazepam), and Tranxene (clorazepate). These drugs are also employed for the treatment of seizures as in delirium tremens.

2. *Antidepressant drugs.* Antidepressant drugs have been used for the treatment of acute and chronic depression since about 1957. Depression that is of recent onset and therefore considered acute can be successfully treated in about 60%–70% of cases. When external circumstances, such as a severe loss, cause the depression, the rate of remission of the depression is not as high. When the depression is endogenous, that is, probably hereditary and lacking any clearly defined external cause, the antidepressants are more effective. A classification of these drugs and their side effects is included in Chapter 14 in this volume.

Before the discovery of the antidepressant drugs, there was no other treatment for serious depression other than electroconvulsive therapy (ECT). This treatment has been viewed with suspicion by the general public. The fear and loathing felt by many stems from the early use of ECT without the simultaneous use of anesthesia. In current ECT treatment, the patient is anesthetized and is unaware of the treatment. In addition, what was formerly a grand mal convulsion following the administration of the treatment is now minor twitching of the fingers, toes, and eyelids. ECT is safe and a highly effective treatment for the chronically depressed or for patients who have not benefited from the antidepressant drugs.

3. *Antipsychotic or neuroleptic drugs.* Antipsychotic and neuroleptic drugs are used mostly in treating the psychoses. In general, they eliminate or ameliorate severe symptoms such as hallucinations (hearing voices or seeing visions), delusions (false beliefs not found in the patient's culture), and severe behavioral disturbances such as homicidal tendencies or other forms of violence. Antipsychotic drugs also are used in calming down the symptoms of manic behavior and the abnormal behavior associated with drug abuse. These drugs do not necessarily lead to a permanent cure, but they have been helpful in allowing many patients to return home and go back to their previous level of functioning. Sometimes the recovery is incomplete, and the patient must remain on the medications for a prolonged time.

4. *Antimanic drugs.* Antimanic drugs are used for the treatment of the manic phase of bipolar disorder. In recent years, it has been shown that drugs such as lithium or Tegretol (carbamazepine) actually can prevent the recurrence of depression or mania in patients who have extremes in mood.

How the Psychiatrist Selects Medications

Emotional and mental disorders can be mild, moderate, or severe. Depending on the severity of the illness, the psychiatrist may elect to prescribe medication or may decide to treat the problem with psychotherapy. If the symptoms are severe, it is important to begin treatment with drugs early. The longer a patient waits to be seen, or the longer the psychiatrist delays treatment, the more difficult it becomes to effect a cure or a remission in symptoms.

Whatever the patient's presenting symptoms are, the psychiatrist uses the drugs that are designed to eliminate the problem. For example, if a patient is severely depressed, the psychiatrist may want to employ an antidepressant that has sedating side effects so that the patient's sleep will be improved while the patient awaits the antidepressant effect of the drug. If the patient is also anxious, a mild tranquilizer could be prescribed as well. On the other hand, if it is necessary that a patient remain fully awake, and he or she is not ill enough to remain away from work, the patient should be given an antidepressant that will not be sedating.

The dose that is prescribed for a given illness differs greatly depending on the severity of the symptoms. Thus, at the beginning of drug administration, the dose may be high, whereas when the patient is partially recovered, the dose may be reduced considerably. Patients receiving medications for chronic conditions almost always receive low doses. Also, each patient tolerates a given drug in his or her own way. Some overreact to most drugs; others need two to three times the amount of medication that is normally given. If there is doubt about how much drug is actually being absorbed into the patient's body, there are standard therapeutic blood levels that have been set for many of the antidepressant and antipsychotic drugs. A psychiatrist may choose to ascertain these levels.

The choice of the proper medication for any disorder is based on certain scientific facts, but using the drugs ultimately is an art that the physician develops. The more experience the physician accumulates, the better the physician will be at selecting the right drug for the symptoms that he or she is attempting to eliminate.

What Can Families, Friends, and Caregivers Do?

Caregivers can be of enormous help to the psychiatrist who is treating a mentally ill person. For example, caregivers can help patients comply with their regular doses of medications. Because of unpleasant side effects of the drugs or because of the mental illness itself (e.g., a paranoid patient may think the drugs are poison), patients do not always want to take prescribed medications. If patients are confused, they may forget to take their medications. Family and friends can be of great assistance in dealing with compliance issues. They can remind the forgetful, coax the reluctant, and make up schedules for the proper times to take medications.

Similarly, caregivers can help patients face their denial of illness. Although not always successful in doing so, those who are close to the patients may help to reinforce the reality of the illness so that the necessary steps can be taken to treat the illness successfully. Friends and family often can motivate patients to do things for themselves, which physicians alone cannot do. The same is true of other caregivers.

Although medications have proven to be of great help in rehabilitating patients, the time it takes for drugs to work is often days to weeks. During this time, much patience is required by the patients as well as the caregivers, and the support of caregivers is most important. For example, an antidepressant drug usually requires several weeks to become effective. While waiting for the drug to become effective, patients are extremely distressed. They need all the support and encouragement they can get to help them through this difficult period.

At other times, patients may become too dependent on medications and not do enough to help themselves. Caregivers can help patients by supporting any suggestions the psychiatrist may make regarding preventing dependence on drugs.

CHAPTER 19

PSYCHOTHERAPY: WHO, WHAT, WHEN, AND HOW?

Psychotherapy is practiced by a number of professionals. Psychiatrists, psychologists, social workers, nurse practitioners, and others do not have equal training, nor are they necessarily trained in psychotherapy. There are minimal standards that everyone who practices psychotherapy must meet, but beyond those, there is much latitude in the training of psychotherapists. Choosing a psychotherapist can be confusing to the person who is just beginning to seek help for an emotional or mental illness.

Most psychologists who practice psychotherapy have a doctorate degree in psychology and have had considerable experience in psychotherapy. Social workers usually have a master's degree in social work and several years of supervised work in psychotherapy before doing psychotherapy on their own.

Credentials and experience are only two measures of a professional's ability to do adequate psychotherapy. For anyone who is seeking help for an emotional or mental illness, I have several suggestions. Perhaps the best way to find a psychotherapist is to ask for a recommendation from a physician, clergyperson, friend, or anyone with whom you have a solid relationship. Upon locating one or two possible therapists, feel free to have a consultation with one or both of these individuals to determine whether you can relate to them. There no doubt are some psychotherapists that you would thoroughly dislike. Overcoming such initial impressions may take a long time and may be unnecessary. Every patient and therapist do not make a good fit. There are times when patients may have to find a second therapist before they feel they can work well with him or her. For those who must go to a clinic setting, such as a community mental health center, the problem is different. You may not have the luxury of being able to choose a psychotherapist; you may be assigned to a therapist. Even in that instance, if there is a personality conflict between you and the therapist, it is not unusual for the treatment team to refer you to another therapist.

In treatment with a psychotherapist, you should be particularly concerned about one important factor: the difficulty of the problem that you have should not be beyond the psychotherapist's competence. For example, a competent psychiatrist who is also a psychoanalyst should not attempt to treat a severe depression with psychoanalysis alone. It is quite likely that even if the treatment went on for considerable time, the depression would not be resolved, a situation that actually happened with one patient as reported in the *Wall Street Journal*. After 2 years of unsuccessful treatment with the psychoanalyst, the patient went to a psychiatrist who was familiar with antidepressants. After only a short interval of treatment with medication, the patient improved and was able to function well again. Of course, a lawsuit followed. Another example is treating patients who have schizophrenia or bipolar disorder without the concomitant use of appropriate medications. Needless to say, other therapists who do not have access to medications when they are indicated should not continue to treat patients indefinitely without resorting to what is known to work.

All too often, someone with limited training tries to treat mentally or emotionally ill persons. There are few laws or rules governing this treatment. For example, a physician not trained in psychiatry could attempt to treat a depressed patient with an antidepressant. The physician may succeed because of the medication, but he or she also may miss the signs of potential suicide in the patient because of a lack of awareness of this possibility. Likewise, a nonmedical psychotherapist is more likely to miss an underlying organic disease that may be responsible for mental or emotional symptoms. Occasionally, I have seen examples of this problem. Good intentions in trying to help the distressed are not enough. The therapist's level of training should match the pathology being treated, or there should be adequate supervision of the therapy by those trained in that specific treatment.

In the course of psychotherapy, if patients have any concern that they are not receiving appropriate treatment, they should consult with another therapist or with a specialist. For example, if persistent headaches and dizziness appear as new symptoms, they should not be dismissed simply as psychologically based. A neurologist should be consulted to rule out any organic disease, such as a brain tumor. Psychotherapists and patients alike should not hesitate to consult with others when they have severe doubts about the course of psychotherapy.

It should be obvious that I do not think that only psychiatrists can do psychotherapy. I know a few psychiatrists to whom I would never refer patients for psychotherapy. These psychiatrists may be good diagnosticians or competent in the use of medications, but they are not psychotherapists. On the other hand, there are certain nonpsychiatrist psychotherapists to whom I gladly refer patients. I judge who is best qualified to help someone based on my experience with these professionals.

Considerations in Starting Therapy

In general, if any of the following six conditions exist, an individual should consult a psychiatrist.

1. *Any psychosis of gradual or sudden onset.* Seeing a psychiatrist when there is a gradual or sudden onset of a psychosis is important. The reason for this recommendation is to rule out

any organic illness that may be the origin of the psychosis. Severe hypertension, hyperthyroidism, brain tumors, and many other organic illnesses can bring about psychoses. A psychiatrist should be aware of the possibility of organic illnesses and properly investigate these illnesses with the help of other specialists.

2. *Bipolar (manic-depressive) disorder.* Both depression and manic behavior can be caused by organic diseases. Physical illness must be ruled out before any attempt is made to do psychotherapy.

3. *Any illness that could be organic and includes many physical symptoms.* In the case of psychosomatic disorders, for which hospitalization of the patient is likely, a psychiatrist would be able to consult with the internist regarding the patient.

4. *Alcoholism or drug abuse with concomitant psychosis, depression, severe anxiety, or gross physical symptoms such as tremors.* When a patient is addicted to alcohol or drugs and has another mental disorder, it is called a dual diagnosis. A competent psychiatrist needs to evaluate and treat patients who have a dual diagnosis.

5. *Doubt about the nature of the illness.* A psychiatrist should be consulted when there is uncertainty about a patient's illness. It also should be emphasized that anyone considering psychotherapy should be examined by a competent family practitioner or internist before starting therapy.

6. *Thoughts of or attempts at suicide.* Anyone who is seriously suicidal should be examined by a psychiatrist first in order to determine whether the person requires hospitalization. Most other mental health professionals are not able to admit patients to a hospital.

Patients who require antidepressants or other psychotropic medications often prefer to be treated by a psychiatrist because a psychiatrist can prescribe medication and do psychotherapy simultaneously. Nonmedical psychotherapists often work closely with psychiatrists in treating the same patient, although the relationship of the two therapists may sometimes be loose and poorly coordinated. It works well for the patient only when the two therapists keep in close contact.

Choosing a Psychotherapy

Psychiatrists and other therapists currently practice many forms of psychotherapy. There are several that are well known and deserve discussion.

Supportive Psychotherapy

Supportive psychotherapy deals directly with a patient's current needs. Although the therapist does take note of the patient's history, he or she does not dwell on it. The therapist tries to keep the therapy on a conscious level, preferring to avoid dealing with dreams or other evidence of unconscious forces. The patient is given advice and reassurance, and alternatives in thinking or behaving are offered. The psychotherapist supports the defenses of the patient when those defenses may be shattered (e.g., in a psychotic disorder). The therapist focuses on symptoms and behaviors rather than the underlying causes of a given disorder. In supportive psychotherapy, the patient's behavior is not interpreted in terms of past life experiences. The therapist may make suggestions, clarify issues, present reality to the patient, and even manipulate the patient's environment to help him or her move on to a healthier state.

Behavioral Psychotherapy

Therapists who practice *behavioral psychotherapy* assume that what has been learned through faulty teaching or adaptation by the individual in his or her early training can be unlearned through behavioral therapy. The therapist is active and directive and assumes the patient will be active in his or her own treatment. The therapy is symptom oriented and does not relate symptoms to past experiences. As with cognitive therapy, in behavioral psychotherapy, patients are given homework to do in between sessions with the therapist. Exposure to feared situations or objects is encouraged through systematic desensitization. For example, in the treatment of a phobia, the patient gradually must try to face the phobia to become desensitized to it.

In behavioral therapy, patients may be exposed to negative or positive reinforcement of their behavior. Negative techniques may even involve aversive procedures such as administering minor shocks to the patient after an undesirable behavior. Positive reinforcement is a reward for altered, desirable behavior. For example, in hospital settings good behavior is rewarded by additional privileges and fewer restrictions. Clearly, the goal is to alter behavior by means of conditioning the patient to unlearn his or her unwanted behaviors and replace them with desirable behaviors.

Cognitive Psychotherapy

Cognitive psychotherapy has some elements in common with behavioral therapy. Both therapies deal with the present and with conscious material; there is no attempt to examine the patient's unconscious or interpret behavior in terms of the past. Those who practice cognitive therapy assume that the patient tells himself or herself negative things throughout the day, which in turn leads to unwanted behaviors and feelings. For example, the altered mood of depression does not come about spontaneously but is due to the intrusion of habitual negative thinking. The cognitive therapist helps the patient become aware of these negative thoughts through homework assignments that identify this undesirable thinking. The patient is asked to compare the typical thoughts with more desirable thoughts, feelings, or behaviors. Gradually, the patient learns to replace negative, emotionally destructive thoughts with positive, ego-enhancing thoughts.

The technique of positive imagery also is used by cognitive therapists. The purposes of this technique are to help elevate the patient's mood and to help the patient experience a heightened sense of enjoyment by envisioning positive and pleasant things consciously and deliberately.

Behavioral and cognitive psychotherapy. *Behavioral* and *cognitive psychotherapy* have a significant place in the treatment of emotional and mental illnesses. These therapies are designed to be of short duration. No effort is made to alter the patient's basic personality traits, but there is an effort to relieve the patient's symptoms and alter behavior. These therapies are sometimes the preferred treatments for certain disorders. Habits such as overeating, smoking, and excessive drinking, as well as phobic disorders, are among the conditions often treated by these methods. Dr. Aaron Beck, author of *Cognitive Theory and the Emotional Disorders*, has been successful in treating mild and moderate depression by means of cognitive therapy.

In addition to the aforementioned therapies, there are other short-term therapies that have been developed. These other therapies include time-limited (12 weeks) therapy, anxiety-provoking therapy, and short-term dynamic psychotherapy. The latter two therapies can last as long as 1 year. Although these therapies are all short-term attempts to help persons with neurotic or personality problems, therapists who practice them accept the theory of the unconscious and the other principles described earlier in this chapter.

Dynamic or Psychoanalytically Oriented Psychotherapy

Dynamic or *psychoanalytically oriented psychotherapy* is designed to be more thorough in reaching the basis of conflicts that bring about emotional illnesses. This type of psychotherapy deals with the present but relates current symptoms and behaviors to the patient's past. It usually is conducted once a week in sessions lasting from 45 to 50 minutes.

The therapy can be short term, but it usually lasts 1–2 years. On occasion, dynamic or psychoanalytically oriented psychotherapy can last even longer if the patient is resistant or the personality problems are severe. For example, Jean, the patient who had borderline personality disorder, described in the case example in Chapter 12, was in treatment for about 3 years. The outcome was favorable, and the patient continued to do well even after many years of follow-up.

Therapists who practice dynamic psychotherapy presume that what happens today in a person's life has antecedents from the patient's past. In an individual's psychological world, history tends to repeat itself. Freud called it repetition-compulsion. In Chapter 12, a case example describes Bethany, who had married and divorced two aggressive men and was married to a third man with similar qualities. She failed to recognize that these men had remarkable similarities to her aggressive but charming father. Upon discovering this repetitious pattern in her life, she was able to make progress toward helping herself work through the problems with her current husband.

Recurring patterns of behavior often are seen in patients who have neuroses and symptoms of depression or anxiety. Failure to express anger and the presence of too much anger that cannot be appropriately expressed are typical examples. Patients who repeatedly cannot express their anger appropriately often are not aware of their pattern of behavior. The goal of therapy is to uncover the patterns and help patients find alternative ways of expressing themselves that are not self-defeating.

In addition, there are some people who constantly find themselves being used. They do not recognize situations in which others are taking advantage of them. In the end, they feel abused, and this feeling leads to low self-esteem and depression. Others repeatedly fail to finish projects because of their perfectionist traits or constantly put off anything someone else wants them to do. These individuals need help in recognizing the patterns that frustrate their progress. Psychotherapy that is psychoanalytically oriented is best suited for this kind of therapeutic work.

What Can Families, Friends, and Caregivers Do?

People frequently ask me, "How can I get my friend or relative to see a psychotherapist?" There is no one answer; however, when someone resists treatment, it helps if the individual first goes to a physician for a physical examination. Perhaps the physician, with a hint from caregivers, will recommend psychotherapy, and this recommendation may be acceptable to the patient.

Sometimes, close friends are more persuasive than family members in getting the person to treatment. Calling upon these friends may be the key to the individual's accepting help.

There are times when family, friends, and other caregivers must wait for a crisis to occur. A sudden panic state, high anxiety, or moderate to severe depression often causes individuals to seek treatment when they previously refused any help. In the case of alcoholic patients, patients addicted to drugs, or pathological gamblers, they often must hit bottom in their personal lives before seeking help for their addiction.

Individuals who develop a psychosis frequently do not realize that they are mentally ill. Family members or close friends first should try to persuade these individuals to go to a psychiatrist voluntarily. Sometimes, however, a legal commitment to a hospital is required. Commitment may be against these patients' will, but it may be necessary so that they receive proper care. At times, it is necessary to call the police to assist with violent or unpredictable behavior.

There is another important aspect to being a caregiver. Some individuals who try to help have a strong feeling that only *they* can really understand and help the person who is emotionally or mentally ill. In psychological jargon, we call this a rescue fantasy. Some caregivers have all-consuming urges to be the one and only person to rescue a patient from his or her problems. I have seen clergy who held on to a congregant much too long before the individual insisted on getting an outside counselor. I have seen friends or neighbors come to the rescue repeatedly when individuals have been in crisis—even suicidal. Instead of calling on the appropriate psychotherapist, they have attempted to handle the problem themselves, being unable to give up the emotional involvement with the patients. Sometimes, these caregivers call on the psychotherapist when it is too late. Caregivers do more good by insisting that the proper help be obtained than by continually trying to help the patients, only to have the crisis and more calls for help recur.

Caregivers occupy an enormous place in helping the emotionally and mentally ill. They are with the patient many more hours than are therapists. Because caregivers play an important role in helping patients, they can consult with the treating psychotherapist if they have the patients' permission. There is little to be gained if the psychotherapist and caregivers are working at cross-purposes. Caregivers have a responsibility to help patients, and the psychotherapist should include caregivers in the treatment whether they are family members, friends, or other professionals.

CHAPTER 20

CONCLUSION

According to the National Institute of Mental Health, there are millions of people who have mental and emotional illnesses:

- More than 11.2 million Americans have depression each year.
- More than 13.3 million adult Americans are afflicted with alcohol abuse or dependence and 5.6 million with drug abuse and dependence.
- More than 2 million Americans are diagnosed as having schizophrenia every year.

Among the anxiety disorders, the following statistics apply:

- Approximately 19.6 million Americans have phobias.
- Approximately 3.8 million Americans have obsessive-compulsive disorder.
- More than 2.3 million Americans have panic symptoms.

Fifty years ago, one-half of all hospital beds in this country were occupied by psychiatric patients. Currently, one-fourth of these beds continue to be occupied by psychiatric patients. This change is one measure of the progress that has been made in treating emotionally and mentally ill patients.

The care of the mentally ill has changed drastically from the exclusive use of hospitals for custodial purposes during the 19th and the beginning of the 20th centuries to rapid treatment via short-term hospitalization and outpatient care. With the birth of psychoanalysis and the beginning of treatment of neurotic disorders with dynamic psychotherapy, the shift to outpatient settings took place. The largest movement occurred with the introduction of mind-altering (psychotropic) drugs. This change enabled many patients to leave the hospital for home or community settings. One of the problems that ensued, unfortunately, was the increase in the homeless population, many of whom are psychiatric patients. Many communities have excellent facilities for the care and housing of the mentally ill. Others are grossly lacking in care and facilities and account for much of the homeless population. Mental health professionals and government officials have yet to solve the problem.

One of the real improvements in the mental health field has been the creation of the small (10–50 beds) psychiatric units in general hospitals. Such facilities are available in many communities for the treatment of acute mental or emotional illnesses. Many patients can now spend less time—a few days to several weeks—on such a unit and return to home and work. Usually, these stays are in conjunction with outpatient care by psychiatrists or other mental health counselors.

Being treated in the general hospital setting has less stigma than being treated in a psychiatric hospital. In addition, the patient's family practitioner, internist, or other specialists are available for consultation. For the psychiatrist, there is the further advantage of being able to consult with these physicians to rule out any organic illnesses that may be causing the mental disturbance. If the patient also has an organic illness, it can be treated simultaneously. Today, helping a patient to recover from an acute illness and return to his or her home or job quickly offers a patient enormous advantages over the state psychiatric hospital routine of 50 years ago.

One of the concerns that has arisen among many psychiatrists is the increasingly short hospital stays required by insurance companies and regulators of health care. In cases of severe mental illness, it takes more than a few days to help a patient over an acute phase of his or her illness so that the patient can at least partially function outside of the hospital. In others cases, such as a patient with a major depression, it takes about 10–15 days for an antidepressant drug to begin to work. More time is required to consolidate the improvement. There are times when insurance companies or managed care providers will demand that patients leave the hospital before they are clinically ready to go. Such conflicts work against the proper care of mentally ill patients. Forced discharge of patients also leads to the revolving-door situation in which patients who are discharged too soon are re-admitted after only a short time outside of the hospital.

Two alternative treatment systems have been developed to address some of these concerns. One is partial hospitalization, in which the patient, after discharge from the hospital, returns to a full- or half-day program for therapy. The other method of treatment is intensive outpatient care, which is used when a patient is acutely ill but not ill enough to warrant admission to a psychiatric unit. Intensive outpatient care also is used when a patient is discharged from the hospital but may need to visit a therapist two to three times per week for individual or group therapy, as well as education about the illness.

Given the enormity of the problem in treating those who are emotionally and mentally ill, mental health professionals need all the help they can get. Whether the person counseling the patient is a psychiatrist, psychologist, social worker, psychiatric nurse, alcohol counselor, activity therapist, psychiatric technician, or other professional counselor, he or she needs help from the patient's caregivers. It cannot be overemphasized that friends, family, and others who are involved in the ongoing daily care of the patient are vitally necessary to the success of any treatment plan that a therapist can devise.

What Can Families, Friends, and Caregivers Do?

In the preceding chapters, I have specified how caregivers can help the emotionally and mentally ill with certain illnesses. To summarize, there are many ways that caregivers can help. Patients need many things. Perhaps the most important of these is the stable, consistent security that family, friends, or other caregivers can provide. In psychiatric jargon, the term is *object constancy*. That is, the caregiver should be the one person on whom the patient can rely. In attempting to help, the caregiver should be dependable, should try to help the patient grow emotionally, should not be too quick to give advice, and should not coerce the patient to do many things against his or her will. Because a mental illness causes confusion daily in the life of the patient, there has to be a reliable base. Although it may be too much to ask the caregiver to be there consistently as the patient's "solid rock," the concept of object constancy is a goal to strive toward rather than an absolute marker in the process of helping the patient heal.

It is important for the caregiver to be as informed as possible on the subject of mental health. I am not suggesting that the caregiver become the patient's therapist; however, basic facts that are helpful to know include a general knowledge of the patient's illness, the therapeutic effects and side effects of medications, and the patient's prognosis.

In addition, caregivers can help by informing the psychiatrist about the patient's full medical history—something that the patient may not always be able to do. Family and friends can remind the patient when to take medication and to be compliant about taking the correct dose. Because many psychotropic drugs do not show their therapeutic effects for days or months, caregivers can remind the patient that feeling better takes time. Also, the patient has to be encouraged to endure side effects if the benefits from the drugs outweigh the disadvantages—as they should.

Communication with the treating psychiatrist or other mental health professional is important for any caregiver. The healing process is difficult when the caregiver and the therapist work at cross-purposes. I am aware that some therapists are not inclined to communicate with relatives or friends of patients. I feel that this lack of communication is a missed opportunity. It is my practice to take all the help I can get in working with patients. Although it does not apply to every patient, I may want to know what is happening at home, whether a patient takes his or her medication regularly, what the caregiver thinks about the patient's progress, and whatever other information is relevant. Information from caregivers is especially helpful in the treatment of the severely mentally ill. A professional working alone cannot get the full picture of how a patient is progressing. If caregivers encounter a psychiatrist who will not cooperate and work directly with them, they should seek another psychiatrist for the patient.

Patients often are not aware that they are developing symptoms of an illness (e.g., the onset of depression or mania). Family and friends can be alert to the beginning of the illness and encourage their relatives or friends to seek help, particularly when the illness recurs.

Patients need a supportive environment to affirm their very existence. I am a small but significant part of that environment; however, I cannot do it alone. Caregivers are essential to providing support and security to patients.

It is important that caregivers not try to change the personality of the patient. It is helpful to recognize the outstanding personality traits that a patient manifests throughout the day, but it is not possible or desirable to try to alter these traits. For example, if the patient has obsessive-compulsive traits and is unusually neat and clean, caregivers should not strive to change those traits in the course of helping him or her overcome a depression, a psychosis, or any other disorder. Rather, caregivers should work around these traits, using them when it would be consistent with the recommended treatment. For example, obsessive-compulsive traits work favorably when caregivers request a patient who has these traits to take prescribed medication at the correct time. The same patient would be upset by not having daily bowel movements or by missing several hours of sleep per night. Caregivers would be wasting time if they tried to persuade the patient that these matters were of no concern. Caregivers must be content with limited goals, which do not include changing the personality of the patient.

Relatives, friends, and other caregivers should be supportive without being a permanent crutch. Many patients can become dependent on caregivers to such an extent that they do not benefit from the interaction. One purpose of caregivers is to help patients grow and become more self-sufficient and strong. Remaining dependent on caregivers may be necessary in certain instances, but whenever possible, dependence should be minimized.

Codependency, a concept discussed in Chapter 8 in this volume, is a term that Alcoholics Anonymous uses. Codependency indicates that caregivers, in their need to help, can become dependent on the patient for the fulfillment of their own needs. Thus, caregivers need the experience and the relationship with the patient as much as the patient needs the help of the caregivers. Professionals, family members, and friends can fall into the trap of needing the patient more than the patient needs them. Codependent caregivers can do more harm than good in helping the patient seek his or her own growth and development. Caregivers in the helping professions should be aware of codependency so as to avoid becoming too dependent on the patient for emotional support.

In Chapter 5 in this volume, I included a list of basic needs common to everyone. Among these are physical, emotional, intellectual, creative, social, and existential needs, as well as the need for recreation and play. Frequently, in the all-encompassing task of giving care to others, helpers neglect their own needs, which is a significant mistake. Caregivers only can be as good as their own physical and emotional health will permit. I have seen family members spend entire days trying to help a distressed patient. For a few days, this continuous help may be necessary and quite possible, but caregivers cannot neglect their own needs. If they repeatedly neglect their own needs, the caregivers will be inadequate and become emotionally disabled themselves. I cannot stress strongly enough that caregivers, whether family, friends, or professionals, have to provide for their own needs or they will be of no use to anyone.

From my own practice, I can provide an example of the effects of ignoring my basic needs. When I first began practicing psychiatry, there were few psychiatrists in my area. I soon was overwhelmed with work. Each time I accepted a new patient, it would mean an additional 1–2 hours a week added to my full schedule. It became especially difficult when a physician friend would call me and ask that I see one of his patients who needed urgent care. When I took on too much work, I became extremely irritable and mildly depressed—overwhelmed. I became less than optimally effective in the work with the patients whom I had already agreed to treat. I soon realized that I had to say no to new patients sometimes if I was going to enjoy my practice and be truly helpful to my patients. Over the years, I have had to remind myself of this basic principle repeatedly.

All caregivers have to work within their limits—physical, emotional, and age limits. Relatives, friends, and other caregivers who help the emotionally or mentally ill are an invaluable source of help. Patients do not live in a vacuum; their environment can help or harm them. The illnesses that humankind must endure, whether mental, emotional, or physical, cannot be treated by professionals alone. We need all the help we can get.

SUGGESTED READINGS

Chapter 1

Eisenstein VW: Neurotic Interaction in Marriage. New York, Basic Books, 1956

Chapter 2

Erikson E: Childhood and Society, 2nd Edition. New York, WW Norton, 1963

Evans RI: Dialogues With Erik Erikson. New York, Harper & Row, 1967

Freud S: The Standard Edition of the Complete Psychological Works of Sigmund Freud, Vols 1–24. Translated and edited by Strachey J. London, Hogarth Press, 1953–1966

Kaplan HI, Sadock BJ, Grebb JA (eds): Kaplan and Sadock's Synopsis of Psychiatry, 7th Edition. Baltimore, MD, Williams & Wilkins, 1994

Spitz RA: The First Year of Life. New York, International Universities Press, 1965

Chapter 3

American Psychiatric Association: Diagnostic and Statistical Manual of Mental Disorders, 4th Edition. Washington, DC, American Psychiatric Association, 1994

Frank LK: Society As the Patient. New Brunswick, NJ, Rutgers University Press, 1950

Goldin LR, Gershon ES: Association and linkage studies of genetic marker loci in major psychiatric disorders. Psychiatric Developments 4:387–418, 1983

Goldman HH: Review of General Psychiatry, 2nd Edition. Norwalk, CT, Appleton & Lange, 1988

Kaplan HI, Sadock BJ, Grebb JA (eds): Kaplan and Sadock's Synopsis of Psychiatry, 7th Edition. Baltimore, MD, Williams & Wilkins, 1994

Rainer JD: Genetics and psychiatry, in Comprehensive Textbook of Psychiatry/IV, 4th Edition, Vol 1. Edited by Kaplan HI, Sadock BJ. Baltimore, MD, Williams & Wilkins, 1985, pp 25–42

Schuckit MA: Genetic and clinical implications of alcoholism and affective disorders. Am J Psychiatry 143:140–147, 1986

Chapter 4

Cousins N: Anatomy of an Illness. New York, Bantam Books, 1981

Cousins N: Head First. New York, EP Dutton, 1989

Hanson PG: The Joy of Stress. Kansas City, MO, Andrews & McMeel, 1986

Selye H: Stress Without Distress. New York, New American Library, 1974

Sullivan HS: Conceptions of Modern Psychiatry. New York, WW Norton, 1947

Chapter 5

Gawain S: Creative Visualization. New York, Bantam, 1985

Hofer E: The True Believer. New York, New American Library, 1951

Hofer E: The Ordeal of Change. New York, Harper & Row, 1963

Kandel ER: Genes, nerve cells, and the remembrance of things past. J Neuropsychiatry Clin Neurosci 1:103–125, 1989

Kaplan HI, Sadock BJ, Grebb JA (eds): Kaplan and Sadock's Synopsis of Psychiatry, 7th Edition. Baltimore, MD, Williams & Wilkins, 1994

Moore T: Care of the Soul: A Guide for Cultivating Depth and Sacredness in Everyday Life. New York, HarperCollins, 1992

Chapter 6

American Psychiatric Association: Diagnostic and Statistical Manual of Mental Disorders, 4th Edition. Washington, DC, American Psychiatric Association, 1994

Andreasen NC, Hoenk PR: The predictive value of adjustment disorders: a follow-up study. Am J Psychiatry 139:584–590, 1982

Klerman GL, Weissman MM: Affective responses to stressful life events. Paper presented at the National Institute of Mental Health Conference on Prevention of Stress-Related Psychiatric Disorders, University of California at San Francisco, December 1981

Chapter 7

American Psychiatric Association: Diagnostic and Statistical Manual of Mental Disorders, 4th Edition. Washington, DC, American Psychiatric Association, 1994

Freud S: The Standard Edition of the Complete Psychological Works of Sigmund Freud, Vol 10. Translated and edited by Strachey J. London, Hogarth Press, 1955

Griest JH, Jefferson JW: Anxiety and Its Treatment: Help Is Available. Washington, DC, American Psychiatric Press, 1986

Horney K: The Neurotic Personality of Our Time. New York, WW Norton, 1947

Schreiber FR: Sybil. New York, Warner Paperback, 1973

Chapter 8

American Psychiatric Association: Diagnostic and Statistical Manual of Mental Disorders, 4th Edition. Washington, DC, American Psychiatric Association, 1994

Beattie M: Codependent No More. San Francisco, CA, Harper & Row, 1987

Kaplan HI, Sadock BJ, Grebb JA (eds): Kaplan and Sadock's Synopsis of Psychiatry, 7th Edition. Baltimore, MD, Williams & Wilkins, 1994

Practice guidelines for the treatment of patients with substance use disorders: alcohol, cocaine, opioids. Am J Psychiatry 152 (suppl):12, 1995

Schuckit MA: Drug and Alcohol Abuse: A Clinical Guide to Diagnosis and Treatment. New York, Plenum, 1979

Smith DE, Gay DR (eds): It's So Good, Don't Even Try It Once. Englewood Cliffs, NJ, Prentice Hall, 1972

Chapter 9

American Psychiatric Association: Diagnostic and Statistical Manual of Mental Disorders, 4th Edition. Washington, DC, American Psychiatric Association, 1994

Gardner R: True and False Accusations of Child Abuse. Cresskill, NJ, Creative Therapeutics, 1992

Kaplan HI, Sadock BJ, Grebb JA (eds): Kaplan and Sadock's Synopsis of Psychiatry, 7th Edition. Baltimore, MD, Williams & Wilkins, 1994

Kaplan HS: Sexual Aversion: Sexual Phobias and Panic Disorders. New York, Brunner/Mazel, 1987

Kaplan LJ: Temptations of Emma Bovary. New York, Doubleday, 1991

Kinsey A, Pomeroy W, Martin CE: Sexual Behavior in the Human Male. Philadelphia, WB Saunders, 1948

Masters WH, Johnson VE: Human Sexual Response, Boston, Little, Brown, 1966

Masters WH, Johnson VE: Human Sexual Inadequacy, Boston, MA, Little, Brown, 1970

Yapko MD: Suggestions of Abuse. New York, Simon & Schuster, 1994

Chapter 10

Agras WS: Eating Disorders: Management of Obesity, Bulimia and Anorexia Nervosa. Oxford, England, Pergamon, 1987

American Psychiatric Association: Diagnostic and Statistical Manual of Mental Disorders, 4th Edition. Washington, DC, American Psychiatric Association, 1994

Bruch H: Eating Disorders: Obesity, Anorexia and the Person Within. New York, Basic Books, 1973

Goldman HH: Review of General Psychiatry, 2nd Edition. Norwalk, CT, Appleton & Lange, 1988

Kaplan HI, Sadock BJ, Grebb JA (eds): Kaplan and Sadock's Synopsis of Psychiatry, 7th Edition. Baltimore, MD, Williams & Wilkins, 1994

Zraly K, Swift D: Anorexia, Bulimia, and Compulsive Overeating. New York, Continuum, 1990

Chapter 11

Bowlby J: Attachment and Loss, Vol 3: Loss, Sadness and Depression. New York, Basic Books, 1980

Freud S: Mourning and melancholia (1917 [1915]), in The Standard Edition of the Complete Psychological Works of Sigmund Freud, Vol 14. Translated and edited by Strachey J. London, Hogarth Press, 1957, pp 237–260

James JW, Cherry F: The Grief Recovery Handbook. New York, HarperCollins, 1989

Kubler-Ross E: On Death and Dying. New York, Macmillan, 1969

Chapter 12

American Psychiatric Association: Diagnostic and Statistical Manual of Mental Disorders, 4th Edition. Washington, DC, American Psychiatric Association, 1994

Edgerton JE, Campbell RJ III (eds): American Psychiatric Glossary, 7th Edition. Washington, DC, American Psychiatric Association, 1994

Johnson SM: Characterological Transformation. New York, WW Norton, 1985

Kernberg O: Borderline Conditions and Pathological Narcissism. New York, Jason Aronson, 1975

Malerstein AJ, Ahern M: A Piagetian Model of Character Structure. New York, Human Sciences Press, 1982

Thomas A, Chess S: Temperament and Development. New York, Brunner/Mazel, 1977

Chapter 13

Goldman HH: Review of General Psychiatry, 2nd Edition. Norwalk, CT, Appleton & Lange, 1988

Kaplan HI, Sadock BJ, Grebb JA (eds): Kaplan and Sadock's Synopsis of Psychiatry, 7th Edition. Baltimore, MD, Williams & Wilkins, 1994

Chapter 14

American Psychiatric Association: Diagnostic and Statistical Manual of Mental Disorders, 4th Edition. Washington, DC, American Psychiatric Association, 1994

Kaplan HI, Sadock BJ: Mood disorders, in Kaplan and Sadock's Synopsis of Psychiatry, 7th Edition. Edited by Kaplan HI, Sadock BJ, Grebb JA. Baltimore, MD, Williams & Wilkins, 1994, pp 516–572

Klerman GL: History and developments of modern concepts of affective illness, in Neurobiology of Mood Disorders. Edited by Post RM, Ballenger JC. Baltimore, MD, Williams & Wilkins, 1984, pp 1–19

Chapter 15

American Psychiatric Association: Diagnostic and Statistical Manual of Mental Disorders, 4th Edition. Washington, DC, American Psychiatric Association, 1994

Arieti S: Interpretation of Schizophrenia, 2nd Edition. New York, Basic Books, 1974

Bleuler E: Dementia Praecox, or the Group of Schizophrenias. New York, International Universities Press, 1950

Goldman HH: Review of General Psychiatry, 2nd Edition. Norwalk, CT, Appleton & Lange, 1988

Greenberg J: I Never Promised You a Rose Garden. New York, Signet, 1964

Kaplan B: The Inner World of Mental Illness. New York, Harper & Row, 1964

Kaplan HI, Sadock BJ, Grebb JA (eds): Kaplan and Sadock's Synopsis of Psychiatry, 7th Edition. Baltimore, MD, Williams & Wilkins, 1994

Kraepelin E: Dementia Praecox. London, ES Livingstone, 1919

Low AA: Mental Health Through Will Training. Glencoe, IL, Willett, 1986

Schneider K: Clinical Psychopathology. New York, Grune & Stratton, 1959

Sullivan HS: Schizophrenia As a Human Process. New York, WW Norton, 1962

Chapter 16

American Psychiatric Association: Diagnostic and Statistical Manual of Mental Disorders, 4th Edition. Washington, DC, American Psychiatric Association, 1994

Cameron NA: Paranoid conditions and paranoia, in American Handbook of Psychiatry, Vol 3. Edited by Arieti S, Brody EB. New York, Basic Books, 1974, pp 676–693

Chapter 17

Lishman WA: Organic Psychiatry, 2nd Edition. Oxford, England, Blackwell Scientific, 1987

Yesavage J: Dementia: differential diagnosis and treatment. Geriatrics 34:51–59, 1979

Yudofsky SC, Hales RE (eds): The American Psychiatric Textbook of Neuropsychiatry, 2nd Edition. Washington, DC, American Psychiatric Press, 1992

Chapter 18

Freud S: The psychopathology of everyday life (1901), in The Standard Edition of the Complete Psychological Works of Sigmund Freud, Vol 6. Translated and edited by Strachey J. London, Hogarth Press, 1960

Freud S: The Ego and the Mechanisms of Defense. New York, International Universities Press, 1946

Maltzer H (ed): Psychopharmacology: The Third Generation of Progress. New York, Raven, 1987

Schatzberg AF, Cole JO: Manual of Clinical Psychopharmacology. Washington, DC, American Psychiatric Press, 1989

Yudofsky SC, Hales RE, Ferguson T: What You Need to Know About Psychiatric Drugs. New York, Grove Weidenfeld, 1991

Chapter 19

Beck AT: Cognitive Theory and the Emotional Disorders. New York, International Universities Press, 1976

Davanloo H (ed): Short-Term Dynamic Psychotherapy. New York, Jason Aronson, 1980

Gabbard GO: Psychodynamic Psychiatry in Clinical Practice: The DSM-IV Edition. Washington, DC, American Psychiatric Press, 1994

Klerman GL, Weissman MM, Rounsaville BJ, et al: Interpersonal Psychotherapy of Depression. New York, Basic Books, 1984

Mann J: Time-Limited Psychotherapy. Cambridge, MA, Harvard University Press, 1973

Novalis PN, Rojcewicz SJ, Peele R: Clinical Manual of Supportive Psychiatry. Washington, DC, American Psychiatric Press, 1993

Sifneos PE: Short-Term Psychotherapy and Emotional Crisis. Cambridge, MA, Harvard University Press, 1972

Ursano RJ, Sonnenberg SM, Lazar SG: Concise Guide to Psychodynamic Psychotherapy. Washington, DC, American Psychiatric Press, 1991

Chapter 20

Korpell HS: How You Can Help: A Guide for Families of Psychiatric Hospital Patients. Washington, DC, American Psychiatric Press, 1984

Additional Readings

Kaplan HI, Sadock BJ (eds): Comprehensive Textbook of Psychiatry/VI, 6th Edition, Vols 1 and 2. Baltimore, MD, Williams & Wilkins, 1995
Stoudmire A: Clinical Psychiatry, 2nd Edition. Philadelphia, JB Lippincott, 1994
Stoudmire A: Human Behavior, 2nd Edition. Philadelphia, JB Lippincott, 1994
Talbott JA, Hales RE, Yudofsky SC (eds): The American Psychiatric Press Textbook of Psychiatry, 2nd Edition. Washington, DC, American Psychiatric Press, 1994

INDEX

Abcesses, of brain, 281
Accidents, and loss of function, 198
Acquired immunodeficiency syndrome (AIDS), 41, 140, 161
Acrophobia, 104
Acting out, 302
Acute stress disorder, 109
Adapin, 246
Adaptation, to loss, 200
Addiction, criteria for, 123–124. See also Drug abuse
Addison's disease, 279
Adjustment disorders, 85–86, 95
Adolescence
  anorexia and, 171
  gender identity disorders and, 145
  modern culture and, 23, 57
  onset of schizophrenia during, 253–254, 255
  as stage in child development, 29
  stress and, 57, 61
Adrenal glands, 52, 279
Adult Children of Alcoholics, 136

Adulthood stage, of life cycle, 30–31
Adults, major stressors for, 62–67
Aesthetics, and creative needs, 75
Age. See also Adolescence; Children; Elderly
  course of schizophrenia and, 255
  depression and age-related peaks in suicide, 237
  distortions in perception of aging process, 168
Aggression and aggressive behavior, 17, 217–218
Agoraphobia
  antidepressants and, 249
  family, friends, and caregivers of patients with, 118
  panic disorders and, 102–103
  stress and child development, 59
Agranulocytosis, 262
Akathisia, 262
Akinesia, 262
Al-Anon, 6, 136
Alateen, 136
Alcoholic intoxication, 127

Alcoholics Anonymous (AA), 6,
11, 12, 78, 123, 125–126,
135, 136, 138, 176
Alcohol-induced disorders, 127
Alcoholism and alcohol abuse
brain function and, 277
child abuse and, 60
as common problem in
psychiatry, 11–12
denial and, 301, 302
dual diagnosis of psychiatric
disorder and, 312
family, friends, and caregivers
for patients with,
137–138
forms of, 127–128
genetics and, 43, 46, 48, 126
patterns of alcohol
consumption, 125
prevalence of, 124–125, 319
reasons for excessive drinking,
125–126
signs of alcohol dependency,
123–124
treatment of, 134–137
Alcohol use disorders, 127
Alcohol withdrawal syndrome,
127
Alcohol withdrawal syndrome
with delirium, 127–128
Allergies, and hives, 94
Alprazolam, 103, 305
Alzheimer's disease, 277, 285
Amenorrhea, 171
American Academy of
Psychiatrists in Alcoholism
and Addictions, 134
American Board of Psychiatry and
Neurology, 292
American Heart Association, 79

American Psychiatric Association,
160. See also Diagnostic and
Statistical Manual of Mental
Disorders
Amitriptyline, 103, 246
Amnesia, 115. See also
Dissociative amnesia
Amnestic disorder, 276
Amoxapine, 246
Amphetamines, 132
Amytal sodium, 108, 111
Anafranil, 105
Anal stage, of psychosexual
development, 24–25
Anger, and loss, 187–188
Animals
research on genetics of
psychiatric illnesses and,
47
sexuality and mating rituals of,
140
Anorexia. See also Eating disorders
body image and, 110, 167–168
case example of, 169–170
causes of, 172
characteristics of, 171
oral stage of development and,
24
recent increase in incidence of,
166–167
sexuality and, 146
treatment of, 173–174
Anorgasmia, 155
Antianxiety drugs, 118, 305
Anticholinergic drugs, 264
Antidepressant drugs. See also
Tricyclic antidepressants
anorexia and, 173
colitis and, 91
depression and, 238

loss and, 201
mechanisms of action, 304
migraine attacks and, 93
overview of use, 305
pain reduction and, 114, 249
panic attacks and, 103, 249
substance abuse and
    depression, 137
Antihistamines, 264
Antihypertension drugs, 153, 155
Antimanic drugs, 304, 306
Antipsychotic drugs
    classification of, 260–261
    mechanisms of action, 260,
        304
    overview of use, 306
    side effects of, 262–264
    treatment of schizophrenia
        with, 261–262, 264–267
Antisocial behavior, 127. *See also*
    Antisocial personality
    disorder; Behavior
Antisocial personality disorder. *See
    also* Antisocial behavior
    characteristics of, 212
    drug abuse and, 133
    interpersonal relationships and,
        64
Anxiety. *See also* Anxiety
    disorders
    alcohol consumption and, 126
    causes of excessive, 18–19
    definition of, 101
    elderly and, 279
    fear of mental illness and, 14
    separation and child
        development, 32
    sexuality and, 155
    stress and, 53
    substance abuse and, 312

temporary excesses in stress
    and, 4
Anxiety disorders. *See also*
    Anxiety
    acute stress disorder, 109
    generalized anxiety disorder,
        109
    genetics of, 46
    obsessive-compulsive disorder,
        105–107
    panic disorder, 101–103
    posttraumatic stress disorder,
        107–108
    prevalence of, 319
    social phobia, 104
    specific phobia, 103–104
    as type of neurosis, 101
Anxiety-provoking therapy, 315
Aquaphobia, 104
Art, and stress management,
    75–76
Artane, 264
Arteriosclerosis, 278, 281
Asendin, 246
Asthma, and stress, 19, 53, 277
Ativan, 305
Atopic dermatitis, 93, 94
Attachment, and development of
    infant, 59
Autonomic nervous system, and
    stress, 53
Aventyl, 246
Avoidance, 103, 104
Avoidant personality disorder,
    213

Barbiturates, 132
Bargaining, and loss, 189–190
Beattie, Melody, 135
Beck, Aaron, 315

Behavior. *See also* Aggression and
    aggressive behavior; Antisocial
    behavior; Personality
dynamic psychotherapy and
    recurring patterns of, 316
influence of genetics on, 35–36,
    37–38
Behavioral psychotherapy,
    313–314, 315
Benadryl, 264
Benztropine, 264
Beriberi, 280
Biochemistry. *See* Brain
Bipolar disorder
    classification of, 242–243
    genetics and, 43, 45–46, 46–47,
        48, 244–245
    normal variations in mood
        versus, 10
    psychotherapy and, 312
    treatment of, 10–11
Bisexuality, 61
Body dysmorphic disorder,
    109–110
Body image, distortions of, 110,
    167–168, 171
Bonding, and development of
    infant, 59
Borderline personality disorder
    brief psychotic disorder and,
        271
    case example of, 218–219
    characteristics of, 212
    duration of psychotherapy for,
        315
Bowel training, and anal stage of
    psychosexual development, 24
Brain, biochemistry and
    physiology of
    alcohol and, 127–128

antipsychotic drugs and, 262
cognitive disorders and,
    277–281
depression and, 238, 246
intermittent explosive disorder
    and injury to, 228
medications and understanding
    of, 303–304
panic disorders and imaging
    studies, 103
schizophrenia and, 45
Brief psychotic disorder, 271
Bulimia. *See also* Eating disorders
    body image distortion and,
        167–168
    case examples of, 175–176
    causes of, 175
    characteristics of, 174
    oral stage of development and,
        24
    recent increase in incidence of,
        166–167
    treatment of, 176

Caffeine, 72, 280
Carbamazepine, 245, 306
Cardiac arrhythmias, and stress,
    53
Caregivers, recommendations for
    helping patients with
    adjustment disorders, 95
    cognitive disorders, 286–288
    common questions asked by, 6
    depression, 249–251
    eating disorders, 181–182
    factitious disorders, 229
    impulse-control disorders,
        229–230
    neuroses, 118–119
    loss, 201–203

obsessive-compulsive disorder,
107
panic disorder, 118
personality disorders,
215–222
phobias, 118, 119
psychiatrists and, 307–308
psychosomatic disorders, 95
psychotherapy and, 316–318
psychotic disorders, 273
schizophrenia, 267–268
sexual disorders, 162
substance abuse, 137–138
summary of, 321–325
*Care of the Soul: A Guide for
Cultivating Depth and
Sacredness in Everyday Life*
(Moore), 75
Case examples
adjustment disorders, 86
anorexia nervosa, 169–170
bulimia, 175–176
cognitive disorders, 276,
284–285
conversion disorder, 110–112
countertransference, 298–299
depression, 9–10, 191–192,
238–241
dissociative amnesia, 116
drug abuse, 129–130
elderly, 13–14
exhibitionism, 150
fear of mental illness, 14
gender identity disorder, 144
loss and depression, 191–192
loss and work issues, 193–194
manic attacks, 244
multiple symptoms, 16
neurosis, 97–99
obesity, 180–181

obsessive-compulsive disorder,
105–107
panic disorder, 7–8
pathological gambling, 226
personality disorders, 205–206,
216, 217–218, 218–219
psychosomatic disorders,
89–90, 91–92, 92–93
schizophrenia, 253–254,
264–265
schizophreniform disorder, 270
stress management, 69–71
transference, 296–297
treatment of sexual disorders,
159
Castration anxiety, 25
Catatonic type, of schizophrenia,
257
Ceci, Stephen, 148
Certification, of psychiatrists,
292–293
Charcot, Jean-Martin, 100
Cherry, Frank, 200–201
Child abuse. *See also* Children
developing child and
experience of sexual
abuse, 147–148
dissociative identity disorder,
116
stress and child development,
59–60
Childbirth, and stress on infant,
58–59
Children. *See also* Adolescence;
Child abuse; Development;
Infant; Parenting
genetics and temperament of,
209–210
history of concepts of
childhood and, 22–23

Children *(continued)*
    influence of on developmental
        environment, 36–37
    sexual abuse and development
        of, 147–148
    stress and development of,
        58–62
Chlordiazepoxide, 305
Chlorpromazine, 173, 260, 261
Chlorprothixene, 261
Civil rights movement, 41
Clomipramine, 105
Clorazepate, 305
Clozapine, 261, 262
Clozaril, 261, 262
Cluster A personality disorders,
        211
Cluster B personality disorders,
        212–213
Cluster C personality disorders,
        213–214
Cocaine, 131, 132
Codependency, and substance
        abuse, 135–136, 324
Codependent No More (Beattie),
        135
Cogentin, 264
Cognitive disorders
    amnestic disorder, 276
    case examples of, 276, 284–286
    delirium, 275
    dementia, 275
    diagnosis of, 281–283
    emotional disorders and,
        284–286
    family, friends, and caregivers
        of patients with, 286–288
    overview of, 277–281
Cognitive psychotherapy, 314–315
Colitis

as psychosomatic illness, 87,
        90–91
    stress and, 19, 53
Colleges, behavioral norms and
        stress, 57
Communes, and cultural change,
        42
Communication, of caregivers
        with mental health
        professionals, 322–323
Community mental health
        centers, and schizophrenia,
        266
Compulsions, definition of, 105
Computed tomography (CT)
        scans, 114, 282, 283
Concordance. *See* Twin studies
Conversion disorder, 110–112
Coprophilia, 152
Countertransference, and
        psychotherapy, 297–299
Creative needs, and mental health,
        75–76
Culture
    adolescence and, 23, 29, 57
    alcoholism and, 125
    anorexia and, 172
    causes of mental illness and,
        40–42
    grief and, 200
    media and children, 48, 58
    nutrition and eating habits, 166
    parenting and changes in,
        42–43
    phobias and phobic disorders,
        8, 9
    prevalence of schizophrenia
        and, 44
    sexuality and, 139, 142–143,
        161–162

stress and, 55–58
Cyclothymic disorder, 242

Death
    sequential separations and life
        cycle, 33–34
    stages of grief in family and,
        190–192
Decision-making, difficulty in, 14,
    15
Defense mechanisms
    loss and, 185–190, 199
    neurotic behavior and, 84
    psychotherapy and, 300–302
Delirium, and cognitive disorders,
    275
Delirium tremens, and
    schizophrenia, 137
Delusional disorder, 271–272
Dementia, 275, 278–281
Denial, 186–187, 301–302
Depakote, 245
Department of Health and
    Human Services, Substance
    Abuse and Mental Health
    Administration, 134
Dependency
    cognitive disorders and,
        287
    oral stage of development and,
        23, 24
Dependent personality disorder,
    213, 220–221
Depersonalization disorder,
    117–118
Depression. *See also* Mood
    disorders
    anorexia and, 173
    cardiac surgery and
        postoperative, 198

case examples of, 9–10,
    191–192, 238–241
classification of, 243
cognitive psychotherapy for,
    314, 315
colitis and, 91
family, friends, and caregivers
    of patients with, 249–251
identification of serious, 234
loss and, 188–189, 198, 201
manic attacks and, 243–245
migraines and, 93
mood versus, 223–234
prevalence of, 236, 319
recognition of, 236–237
sexuality and, 153–154
substance abuse and, 126, 137,
    312
treatment of, 237, 240, 305
types of, 237–241
Depressive neurosis. *See*
    Dysthymic disorder
Desipramine, 246
Desyrel, 249
Development, human. *See also*
    Adolescence; Children; Life
    cycle
    Erickson's eight stages of,
        26–31
    Freud's psychosexual stages of,
        23–26
    influence of children on
        environment for, 36–37
    nutrition and eating habits,
        164–165
    overview of normal, 22–23
    parenting and, 48
    sequential separations and,
        31–34
    sexual needs and, 140

Diabetes
    brain function and, 278, 279
    obesity and, 179
    sexuality and, 153, 154, 155
Diagnostic and Statistical Manual
    of Mental Disorders, 4th
    Edition (DSM-IV)
    classification of
        bipolar disorder, 45
        disorders due to alcohol, 127
        eating disorders, 168
        mood disorders, 241–243
        neuroses, 100–101
        personality disorders, 211
        psychotic disorders, 269
    criteria for substance
        dependence, 123–124
    definition of anorexia, 171
    description of paraphilias, 146
    obesity as eating disorder and,
        165, 169
    subdivisions of
        adjustment disorders in, 85
        of schizophrenia, 257–259
        of sexual disorders, 156
Diazepam, 305
Diethylpropion, 179
Dieting, and treatment of obesity,
    179, 181
Difficult child, as temperament
    type, 209
Diphenhydramine, 264
Disease and illness. *See also*
    Diabetes; Health; Heart
    disease; Psychosomatic
    disorders
    alcoholism as, 11, 125, 134
    anxiety and, 19
    cognitive disorders and,
        279–281

stress and, 19, 66–67
Disorganized type, of
    schizophrenia, 258
Dissociative amnesia, 116–117.
    See also Amnesia
Dissociative disorders
    depersonalization disorder,
        117–118
    dissociative amnesia, 116–117
    dissociative fugue, 117
    dissociative identity disorder,
        115–116
    symptoms of, 115
    as type of neurosis, 101
Dissociative fugue, 117
Dissociative identity disorder,
    115–116
Divalproex sodium, 245
Divorce. *See also* Marriage
    loss and, 195
    stress and developing child, 60
Dix, Dorothea, 259
Dopamine, and schizophrenia,
    260
Dosages, of tricyclic
    antidepressants, 246
Doxepin, 246
Drug abuse
    case example of, 129–130
    child abuse and, 60
    cognitive disorders and, 278
    as common problem in
        psychiatry, 11–12
    comorbidity of with alcoholism,
        124
    criteria for substance
        dependence, 123–124
    culture and, 40
    dual diagnosis of psychiatric
        disorder and, 312

family, friends, and caregivers
    of patients with, 137–138
personality and, 133–134
prevalence of, 130–132, 319
treatment of, 134–137
Drug interactions, and cognitive
    disorders, 278
Drugs, psychiatric. *See*
    Medications
Dual diagnosis, of substance abuse
    and psychiatric disorder,
    136–137, 312
Dynamic psychotherapy, 315–316
Dyspareunia, 156
Dysthymic disorder, 243
Dystonia, 262

Ears, cognitive disorders and
    diseases of, 280
Eating disorders. *See also*
    Anorexia; Bulimia
classification of, 168–169
family, friends, and caregivers
        of patients with, 181–182
obesity and, 176–181
overview of, 165–168
Economics, and societal cost of
    substance abuse, 124, 132
Eczema, 93, 94
Education
    intellectual needs and good
        mental health, 74
    of psychiatrists, 291–293
    schizophrenia and, 266
    treatment of sexual disorders
        and, 158
Elavil, 103, 246
Elderly
    cognitive disorders and, 279,
        280, 287–288

common problems in
    psychiatry and, 13–14
dosages of medications and,
    246
Erikson's model of life cycle
    and, 31
hearing and vision loss in, 280
loss and depression, 192
monitoring of medication use
    by, 133
nutrition and, 280
sexuality and, 155
social needs of, 77
Electroconvulsive therapy (ECT),
    201, 245, 305–306
Emotional illness, compared with
    mental illness, 83–84. *See also*
    Cognitive disorders; Neuroses
Emotional needs, and good mental
    health, 73–74
Empathy, and care of patients
    with panic disorder, 103
Emphysema, 281
Enablers, and substance abuse,
    134–135, 136
Encephalitis, 281
Endocarditis, 281
Endocrine system and endocrine
    disorders
    cognitive disorders and, 279
    female sexual arousal disorder
        and, 154
    male erectile disorder and, 155
    stress and, 52
Endogenous depression, 238,
    240–241
Epilepsy, 228
Erhard Seminars Training (EST),
    42
Erikson, Erik, 26–31

Ethnicity, and obesity, 177
Exercise
    anorexia and, 171
    anxiety and, 18–19
    family, friends, and caregivers
        of patients and, 119
    obesity and, 179–180
    physical needs and, 72–73
    stress and, 55–56, 79
Exhibitionism, 149–150, 157
Existential needs, and good mental
    health, 77–79
Exogenous depression, 238–240
Eyes, cognitive disorders and
    diseases of, 280

Factitious disorder
    family, friends, and caregivers
        of patients with, 229–230
    with physical symptoms,
        223–224
    with psychological symptoms,
        224–225
Family. See also Marriage;
    Parenting
    anorexia and, 172
    grief and, 190–192
    monitoring of prescription
        medication use, 133
    obsessive-compulsive disorder
        and, 107
    personality disorders and, 17
    recommendations for as
        caregivers of mentally ill
        adjustment disorders and,
            95
        cognitive disorders and,
            286–288
        common questions asked by,
            6

depression and, 234,
    249–251
eating disorders and,
    181–182
factitious disorders and, 229
impulse-control disorders
    and, 229–230
loss and, 201–203
neuroses and, 118–119
panic disorder and, 103, 118
personality disorders and,
    215–222
phobias and, 118, 119
psychiatrists and, 307–308
psychosomatic disorders and,
    95
psychotherapy and, 316–318
psychotic disorders and, 273
schizophrenia and, 266,
    267–268
sexual disorders and, 162
substance abuse and,
    137–138
summary of
    recommendations for,
        321–325
sexual revolution and, 41
Family therapy, for anorexia, 173
Fantasy, and paraphilias, 146. See
    also Rescue fantasies
Fat cell theory, 178
Fear, and stress, 53
Female orgasmic disorder, 155
Female sexual arousal disorder,
    154
Fenfluramine, 179
Fetal alcohol syndrome, 58, 128
Fetishism, 149
Fight or flight reaction, 53
Finances, and stress, 65–66

Flattened affect, in schizophrenia, 255
Fluoxetine, 105, 176, 248
Free association, 100
Freud, Sigmund
  on culture and sexuality, 142
  on development of neuroses, 83–84, 100, 112, 161, 300
  on genetics and behavior, 37–38
  influence of on modern psychiatry, 5, 208
  on loss and depression, 185, 188
  on obesity, 177
  on psychosexual stages of development, 23–26
  on pyromania, 227
  theory of unconscious and, 293, 294
  transference and analytic method of, 295
Friends, recommendations for care of mentally ill by. *See also* Interpersonal relationships
  adjustment disorders and, 95
  cognitive disorders and, 286–288
  common questions asked by, 6
  depression and, 234, 249–251
  eating disorders and, 181–182
  factitious disorders and, 229
  impulse-control disorders and, 229–230
  loss and, 201–203
  neuroses and, 118–119
  obsessive-compulsive disorder and, 107
  panic disorder and, 103, 118

  personality disorders and, 215–222
  phobias and, 118, 119
  psychiatrists and, 307–308
  psychosomatic disorders and, 95
  psychotherapy and, 316–318
  psychotic disorders and, 273
  schizophrenia and, 267–268
  sexual disorders and, 162
  substance abuse and, 137–138
  summary of, 321–325
Frotteurism, 152
Function, loss of, 197–199

Gamblers Anonymous (GA), 226
Gambling, and stress, 65–66. *See also* Pathological gambling
Gardner, Richard, 148
Gender identity disorders, 143–145, 162
Generalized anxiety disorder, 109
Genetic counseling, and psychiatric illnesses, 46–47
Genetics
  alcoholism and, 46, 48, 126
  anxiety disorders and, 46
  bipolar disorder and, 45–46, 46–47, 48, 244–245
  counseling on psychiatric illnesses and, 46–47
  depression and, 238
  homosexuality and, 161
  influence of on behavior, 35–36, 37–38
  mental illness and, 43–47
  obesity and, 177
  panic disorder and, 46
  personality formation and, 208–210

Genetics *(continued)*
  research on genetic markers for
    psychiatric illnesses, 47
  schizophrenia and, 44–45, 48,
    256
Genital stage, of psychosexual
    development, 25–26
Greenberg, Joanne, 265
Grief, 190–192, 200. *See also* Loss
Grief Recovery Handbook, The
    (James & Cherry), 200–201
Group therapy, for posttraumatic
    stress disorder, 108
Growth. *See* Development, human
Guilt
  depression and, 236–237, 250
  masturbation and, 159–160
  paraphilias and, 146
  parenting and, 39

Haldol, 173, 260, 261
Haloperidol, 173, 260, 261
Hand washing, compulsive, 105
Headaches
  brain tumors and, 279, 281
  psychosomatic disorders and,
    91–93
  stress and, 19
Head trauma, and cognitive
    disorders, 280
Health. *See also* Disease and
    illness; Mental health;
    Psychosomatic disorders
  evaluation of before starting
    psychotherapy, 312
  obesity and, 178–179
  psychiatric problems in elderly
    and, 13–14
  sexual desire and, 153, 154
  stress and, 52–53, 64–65

Health care system, and present
    status of mental health care,
    319–321
Heart disease
  alcohol abuse and, 11
  cardiac surgery and loss of
    function, 198–199
  obesity and, 179
  personality and, 88
  sexual desire and, 153
Hepatitis, 262
Heredity. *See* Genetics
History
  of psychiatry, 5, 25, 26, 35–36,
    37–38, 40–42
  of schizophrenia, 259–260
  of views of mental illness, 4–5
Histrionic personality disorder
  brief psychotic disorder and,
    271
  case example of, 216, 221
  characteristics of, 212–213
Hives, 93
Hofer, Eric, 74
Homelessness, and care of
    mentally ill, 320
Homosexuality, 61, 160–161
Hope, and child development, 27
Hormones. *See* Endocrine system
Horney, Karen, 101
Hospitals
  insurance companies and length
    of stay in, 320–321
  legal commitment to, 317
  small psychiatric units in
    general, 320
  state institutions for mentally
    ill, 5
Hydrocortisone, 94
Hyperglycemia, 280

Hyperinsulinism, 179
Hyperthyroidism, 19, 109, 276, 279
Hypnotic drugs, 132
Hypoactive sexual desire disorder, 153–154
Hypochondriasis, 64–65, 113
Hypoglycemia, 19, 109, 279, 280
Hypomania, definition of, 235, 242
Hypothalamus, 52
Hypothyroidism, 154, 276, 279
Hysterical conversion, 100

Identity
    adolescence and formation of, 29
    adolescence and sexual as source of stress, 61
    dissociative fugue, 117
Imipramine, 103, 246
Impotence, 70–71, 154–155
Impulse-control disorders
    characteristics of, 225–226
    family, friends, and caregivers of patients with, 229–230
    intermittent explosive disorder, 228
    kleptomania, 227–228
    pathological gambling, 226
    pyromania, 227
Independence, and loss, 197
I Never Promised You a Rose Garden (Greenberg), 265
Infant, stress and development of, 59. *See also* Children
Infection, and cognitive disorders, 281
Insurance companies, and length of stay in hospital, 320–321

Intellectualization, as defense mechanism, 301
Intellectual needs, and good mental health, 74–75
Intensive outpatient care, 321
Intermittent explosive disorder, 228, 229–230
Interpersonal relationships, and stress, 64. *See also* Family; Friends; Marriage; Social needs
Isocarboxazid, 247
Italy, prevalence of alcoholism in, 125

James, John W., 200–201
Japan, prevalence of alcoholism in, 125
Johnson, Virginia, 158, 159

Kaplan, Louise J., 146
Kleptomania, 227–228, 229
Kline, Nathan, 259
Kubler-Ross, Elisabeth, 186

Laing, R. D., 41
Lamaze method, 118
Latency stage, of child development, 25, 28
Learning, stress and child development, 60
Leary, Timothy, 131
Levothyroxine, 276
Librium, 305
Life cycle, and sequential separations, 31–34. *See also* Development, human
LifeSpring, 42
Lifestyle, and obesity, 180–181

Lithium, 11, 45, 241, 245, 306
Liver disease, 125, 262
Locomotor-genital stage, of child
    development, 28
Lorazepam, 305
Loss. *See also* Grief
    cognitive disorders and, 287
    as common problem in
        psychiatry, 17
    dealing with, 199–201
    defenses against, 185–190
    depression and, 237–240
    divorce and, 195
    families, friends, and caregivers
        of patients with, 201–203
    function and, 197–199
    independence and, 197
    possessions and, 197
    power and, 195–196
    security and, 195
    sequential separations and life
        cycle, 33–34
    sexuality and, 154
    stress and, 66–67
    variations in personal
        experience of, 183–185
    work issues and, 193–194
Low, Abraham, 266
Loxapine, 261
Loxitane, 261
Ludiomil, 249

Magnetic resonance imaging
    (MRI), 282–283
Major depressive disorder, 243
Male erectile disorder, 154–155
Male orgasmic disorder, 155
Malingering, 225
Mania
    definition of, 235

depression and attacks of,
    243–245
family, friends, and caregivers
    of patients with, 250–251
neurotransmitters in brain and,
    246
Manic-depressive disorder. *See*
    Bipolar disorder
Maprotiline, 249
Marijuana, 131–132
Marplan, 247
Marriage. *See also* Divorce
    changes in as common problem
        in psychiatry, 12–13
    denial and problems in, 302
    sequential separations and life
        cycle, 33
    sexual needs and, 140–141
Masochism, 151–152
Masters, William, 158, 159
Masturbation, 159–160
Media, and modern culture, 48,
    58
Medications, psychiatric. *See also*
    Antidepressants;
    Antipsychotic drugs; Dosage;
    Side effects;
    Treatment
    anorexia and, 173
    common questions about use of
        prescribed, 12
    compliance with regimens of,
        322, 323
    drug abuse and prescription,
        132–133
    drug interactions and cognitive
        disorders, 278
    family, friends, and caregivers
        of mentally ill and
        monitoring of, 118–119

mood disorders and, 245–249
obesity and, 179
overview of, 303–306
panic disorders and, 103
psychoses and, 15
research on, 16
schizophrenia and compliance
  problems, 267
selection of by psychiatrist,
  306–307
stress management and, 80
Mellaril, 261
Meningioma, 281
Meningitis, 281
Mental health, basic needs for
  good, 71–79. *See also* Mental
  illness
*Mental Health Through Will
  Training* (Low), 266
Mental illness. *See also* specific
  disorders
comorbidity with substance
  abuse, 132, 136–137
culture as cause of, 40–42
emotional illness compared
  with, 83–84
fear of, 14–15
genetics and, 43–47
health care system and present
  status of care for,
  319–321
history of views of, 4–5
loss of function and, 197–198
prevalence of, 319
stigma of, 5
Mentoring, and adult life, 62
Mesoridazine, 261
Metabolism, and obesity, 177
Methylphenidate, 132
Microphobia, 104

Migraines, 91, 92–93
Minerals, dietary, 72
Moban, 261
Molindone, 261
Monoamine oxidase inhibitors
  (MAOIs), 247–248
Mood, and depression, 233–234,
  235
Mood disorders. *See also*
  Depression
classification of, 241–243
as common problem in
  psychiatry, 9–11
family, friends, and caregivers
  of patients with, 249–251
medications for, 245–249
Moore, Thomas, 75
Mothers, and
  obsessive-compulsive disorder,
  105–107. *See also* Parenting
Multiple personality. *See*
  Dissociative identity disorder;
  Split personality
Munchausen syndrome, 223–224,
  225
Muscular-anal stage, of child
  development, 27–28
Mysophilia, 152
Mysophobia, 104

Narcissistic personality disorder
  characteristics of, 213
  general example of, 219–220
  interpersonal relationships and,
    64
Narcotics Anonymous (NA), 12,
  130, 136, 138
Nardil, 103, 247
National Alliance for the Mentally
  Ill (NAMI), 266, 267

National Institute on Drug Abuse, 131
National Institute of Mental Health (NIMH), 44–45, 126
Navane, 173, 261
Necrophilia, 153
Neurodermatitis. *See also* Skin diseases
  as psychosomatic disorder, 93, 94
  stress and, 19, 53
Neuroleptic drugs. *See* Antipsychotic drugs
Neuroleptic malignant syndrome, 263
Neurological disorders, and sexuality, 153, 154, 155
Neurosis
  acute versus chronic, 84
  case example of, 97–99
  causes of, 99–100
  characteristics of, 83
  defense mechanisms and, 300
  personality disorders compared with, 208
  types of, 100–101
Neurotic interactions, in marriage, 12
Norpramin, 246
North Atlantic Treaty Organization (NATO), 41
Nortriptyline, 246
Nutrition
  cognitive disorders and, 280
  development and, 164–165
  eating habits and, 166
  emotional factors and, 72
  family, friends, and caregivers of patients and, 119
  stress management and, 79

Obesity, 24, 165, 176–181
Object constancy, 322
Obsessions, definition of, 105
Obsessive-compulsive disorders
  anal stage of psychosexual development and, 25
  characteristics of, 105–107, 208, 213–214, 215
  oral stage of psychosexual development and, 23
  prevalence of, 319
  selective serotonin reuptake inhibitors and, 249
  treatment of, 105–107
Oedipal stage, of psychosexual development, 25
Old age and maturity stage, of life cycle, 31
On Death and Dying (Kubler-Ross), 186
Oral-sensory stage, of child development, 26–27
Oral stage, of psychosexual development, 23–24
Organic brain disorders. *See* Cognitive disorders
Orgasmic disorders, 155–156
Overeaters Anonymous, 179

Pain. *See also* Pain disorder
  abuse of prescription medications for, 133
  antidepressants and, 114, 249
  stress and, 19
Pain disorder, 113–115. *See also* Pain
Pamelor, 246
Panic and panic attacks. *See also* Panic disorders
  antidepressants and, 103, 249

prevalence of, 319
stress and, 53–54
Panic disorders. *See also* Panic and
   panic attacks
   case examples of, 7–8
   characteristics of, 101–103
   genetics of, 46
Paranoia. *See* Delusional disorder
Paranoid personality disorder, 17,
   211
Paranoid type, of schizophrenia,
   257–258
Paraphilias
   child abuse and, 60
   definition of, 145
   exhibitionism, 149–150
   fetishism, 149
   frotteurism, 152
   paraphilia not otherwise
      specified, 152–153
   pedophilia, 146–149
   sexual masochism, 151–152
   sexual sadism, 150–151
   treatment of, 156–157, 162
   types of, 145–146
   voyeurism, 152
Parathyroid disease, 279
Parenting. *See also* Children;
   Family; Mothers
   anorexia and, 172
   cultural change and, 42–43
   eating habits and nutrition,
      166
   guilt and, 39
   importance of effective, 48
   schizophrenia and, 43–44
   temperament of child and, 210
Parkinson's disease, 155
Paroxetine, 248
Partial hospitalization, 321

Passive-aggressive personality
   disorder, 206–207
Pathological gambling, 226, 229.
   See also Gambling
Paxil, 248
Pedophilia, 146–149
Peers, and eating habits, 166
Pellagra, 280
Penis envy, 25
Perphenazine, 261
Personality. *See also* Behavior;
   Personality disorders
   drug abuse and, 133–134
   formation of, 208–211
   psychosomatic illnesses and, 88
Personality disorders. *See also*
   Personality
   case examples of, 205–206,
      216, 218–219
   child abuse and, 60
   classification of, 211–214
   as common problem in
      psychiatry, 17–18
   definition of, 207–208
   drug abuse and, 133
   family, friends, and caregivers
      of patients with, 215–222
   interpersonal relationships and,
      64
   psychiatrists and, 214
Pertofrane, 246
Phallic stage, of psychosexual
   development, 25
Phenelzine, 103
Phobias and phobic disorders
   behavioral therapy for, 314
   as common problem in
      psychiatry, 8–9
   family, friends, and caregivers
      of patients with, 118, 119

Phobias and phobic disorders
(continued)
prevalence of, 319
school phobia, 32
social phobia, 104
specific phobias, 103–104
Physical needs, and good mental
health, 71–73
Physiology, and theories on
obesity, 178
Pinel, Philippe, 259
Pituitary gland, 52, 279
Pneumoencephalography, 282
Polysubstance abuse, 132
Pondimin, 179
Positive imagery, and cognitive
therapy, 314
Positron emission tomography
(PET), 283
Posttraumatic stress disorder,
107–108
Power, and loss, 195–196
Pregnancy, stress and fetal
development during, 58
Premature ejaculation, 16,
155–156
Prescription medications
cognitive disorders and
interactions among, 278
common questions concerning,
12
drug abuse and, 132–133
Primary neurosis, 100
Projection, as defense mechanism,
301
Prostate disease, 155
Protriptyline, 246
Prozac, 105, 176, 248
Pseudodementia, 279
Pseudoparkinsonism, 263

Psychiatrists. *See also* Psychiatry
assessment of stress by, 4
competence of in
psychotherapy, 311
family, friends, and caregivers
of patients and, 6,
307–308
personality disorders and, 214
selection of medications by,
306–307
stages of human development
and, 34
training of, 291–293
Psychiatry. *See also* Psychiatrists;
Psychotherapy; Treatment
common problems in
elderly, 13–14
fear of mental illness, 14–15
loss, 17
marriage, 12–13
mood disorders, 9–11
multiple symptoms, 16
panic disorder, 7–8
personality disorders, 17–18
phobic disorders, 8–9
psychoses, 15–16
stress, 18–19
genetics and influence on
behavior, 35–36, 37–38
history of, 5, 25, 26, 35–36,
37–38, 40–42
Psychic determinism, 294
Psychic numbing, 108
Psychoanalysis, of psychiatrists as
part of training, 293, 299
Psychoanalytically oriented
psychotherapy. *See* Dynamic
psychotherapy
Psychopharmacology. *See*
Medication

Psychosexual stages of
   development, 23–26
Psychosis and psychotic disorders.
   See also Schizophrenia
   acute versus chronic, 84
   brief psychotic disorder, 271
   as common problem in
      psychiatry, 15–16
   delusional disorder, 271–272
   emotional disorders compared
      with, 84
   family, friends, and caregivers
      of patients with, 273
   gradual versus sudden onset of,
      311–312
   schizoaffective disorder, 271
   schizophreniform disorder,
      269–270
   shared psychotic disorder,
      272
   substance abuse and, 312
   treatment of, 272–273
Psychosomatic disorders
   characteristics of, 87–88
   colitis, 90–91
   evaluation of health of patient,
      312
   family, friends, and caregivers
      for patients with, 95
   headaches, 91–93
   skin diseases, 93–95
   stomach and duodenal ulcers,
      89–90
Psychotherapy. *See also* Psychiatry;
   Treatment
   basic theoretical assumptions of
      dynamic, 293–302
   choice of forms of, 313–316
   choice of therapist for,
      309–310

   considerations in starting,
      311–313
   evaluation of competence of
      therapist, 310–311
   family, friends, and caregivers
      of patients and, 316–318
   training of psychiatrists in, 292
Pyromania, 227, 229
Pyrophobia, 104

Quiet child, as temperament type,
   209

Rationalization, as defense
   mechanism, 300–301
Recovery (self-help group), 266
Regression, as defense mechanism,
   301
Relapse, of schizophrenia, 265
Relationships. *See* Family; Friends;
   Interpersonal relationships;
   Marriage
Relaxation therapy, and stress
   management, 79–80
Religion, and existential needs,
   77–78
Repetition-compulsion, as pattern
   of behavior, 26
Repression, 84, 300
Rescue fantasies, 202, 317
Reserpine, 259–260
Residency training, of
   psychiatrists, 292
Residual type, of schizophrenia,
   258–259
Resistance, and psychotherapy,
   294–295
Resolution, and loss, 190
Retirement, and loss, 193–194
Risperdal, 261

Risperidone, 261
Ritalin, 132
Role models, and adolescence, 62
Rush, Benjamin, 4–5, 259
Russia, and cultural change in
    1990s, 41

Sadism, 151
Schizoaffective disorder, 271
Schizoid personality disorder, 17,
    211
Schizophrenia. *See also* Psychosis
    and psychotic disorders
    antipsychotic drugs and,
        260–267
    case examples of, 253–254,
        264–265
    causes of, 256–257
    characteristics of, 255
    child abuse and, 60
    as chronic disorder, 84
    course of, 255–256
    definition of, 254–255
    delirium tremens and, 137
    family, friends, and caregivers
        of patients with, 267–268
    genetics and, 43, 44–45, 48,
        256
    history of, 259–260
    parenting and, 43–44
    prevalence of, 15, 256, 319
    regression and, 301
    schizophreniform disorder
        distinguished from, 270
    split personality and, 14–15
    types of, 15, 257–259
Schizophreniform disorder,
    269–270
Schizotypal personality disorder,
    211

School phobia, 32, 59, 102, 195
Scurvy, 280
Seasonal depression and seasonal
    affective disorder, 238, 243
Security, and loss, 195
Selective serotonin reuptake
    inhibitors (SSRIs), 248–249
Self-esteem, and interpersonal
    relationships, 64
Self-help groups. *See also*
    Alcoholics Anonymous;
    Narcotics Anonymous;
    Support groups
    for drug abuse and alcoholism,
        12, 136, 138
    for grief, 200
    for schizophrenia, 266
    for temporary excesses in stress
        and anxiety, 4
Selye, Hans, 52, 53
Sensate focusing, 158
Separation
    human development and,
        31–34
    stress and, 59
Separation anxiety, 32, 59, 102
Sequential separations, and human
    development, 31–34
Serentil, 261
Sertraline, 248
Set point theory, on obesity, 178
Sexual arousal disorders, 154–155
Sexual aversion disorder, 154
Sexual desire disorders, 153–154
Sexual dysfunction. *See also*
    Sexuality
    case example of, 16, 70–71
    orgasmic disorders, 155–156
    sexual arousal disorders,
        154–155

sexual aversion disorder, 154
sexual desire disorders, 153–154
sexual dysfunction due to general medical condition, 156
sexual pain disorders, 156
stress and, 70–71
treatment of, 157–158, 162
Sexuality. *See also* Sexual dysfunction
adolescents and stress, 61
anorexia and, 172
family, friends, and caregivers for patients with disorders related to, 162
gender identity disorders, 143–145
masturbation and sexual orientation distress, 159–161
modern culture and, 40–41, 139, 142–143, 161–162
paraphilias, 145–153
treatment of disorders related to, 156–159
variations in needs, 139–141
Sexual masochism, 151–152
Sexual orientation distress, 160–161
Sexual pain disorders, 156
Sexual sadism, 150–151
Shared psychotic disorder, 272
Shiverer mouse, 47
Short-term psychotherapy, 315
Side effects
of antipsychotic drugs, 262–264
of clozapine, 262
of monoamine oxidase inhibitors, 247–248
of selective serotonin reuptake inhibitors, 249
of tricyclic antidepressants, 246
Sinequan, 246
Single photon emission computed tomography (SPECT), 283
Skin diseases, as psychosomatic illnesses, 87, 93–95. *See also* Neurodermatitis
Sleep, and stress management, 79
Slow to warm up child, as temperament type, 209
Social needs, and good mental health, 76–77. *See also* Interpersonal relationships
Social phobia, 104
Social skills, stress and child development, 60
Society. *See* Culture
Somatization disorder, 112–113
Somatoform disorders
body dysmorphic disorder, 109–110
conversion disorder, 110–112
hypochondriasis, 113
pain disorder, 113–115
somatization disorder, 112–113
as type of neurosis, 101
Spastic colitis, 90
Specific phobias, 103–104
Spinal fluid testing, 282
Spinal myelogram, 114
Split personality, and schizophrenia, 14–15
Splitting, and schizophrenia, 255
Stelazine, 261
Steroids, 278

Stress
  adjustment reactions and, 85
  adults and major sources of,
    62–67
  common problems in
    psychiatry and, 18–19
  definition of, 52
  developing child and, 58–62
  dissociative fugue, 117
  eczema and, 94
  fear, anxiety, and panic, 53–54
  health effects of, 52–53, 87,
    93–94, 276–277
  hives and, 93–94
  management of, 69–71, 79–80
  modern culture and, 55–58
  neurodermatitis and, 94
  normal variations in, 3
  physical symptoms due to,
    276–277
  psychosomatic illnesses and, 87
  temporary excesses in, 3–4
Stress Without Distress (Selye), 52
Sublimation, as defense
  mechanism, 300
Substance abuse. *See* Alcoholism
  and alcohol abuse; Drug abuse
Substance-induced anxiety
  disorder, 109
Substance-induced mood disorder,
  243
Substance-induced sexual
  dysfunction, 156
Suggestions of Abuse (Ceci), 148
Suicide and suicidal ideation
  anorexia and, 171
  depression and, 10, 234, 237,
    250
  loss and, 17, 188–189, 202–203
  psychotherapy and, 312

Sullivan, Harry Stack, 29–30, 64,
  164
Support groups. *See also* Self-help
  groups
  for anorexia, 174
  for schizophrenia, 267
Supportive psychotherapy, 313
Surgery
  cardiac and depression due to
    loss of function, 198–199
  for treatment of obesity, 180
Symptoms, of mental illness
  dissociative disorders and, 115
  multiple forms of as common
    problem in psychiatry, 16
  neuroses versus personality
    disorders, 208
  schizophrenia and, 255
  stress and psychosomatic, 19,
    276–277
  substance abuse and, 123–124
Synthroid, 276
Szasz, Thomas, 41

Taractan, 261
Tardive dyskinesia, 263
Tegretol, 245, 306
Telephone scatologia, 152
Television, 48, 58
Temptations of Emma Bovary
  (Kaplan), 146
Tenuate, 179
Thioridazine, 261
Thiothixene, 173, 261
Thorazine, 173, 260, 261
Thought disorder, schizophrenia
  as, 255
Thyroid disease, and stress, 19, 52
Time-limited therapy, 315
Time management, and stress, 80

Tofranil, 103, 246
Toilet training, and psychosexual development, 24
Tolerance, and substance abuse, 123
Tough Love (self-help group), 42
Tranquilizers, 132, 133
Transference, and psychotherapy, 295–297
Transsexualism, 144
Transvestic fetishism, 149
Tranxene, 305
Travel, and stress, 56
Trazodone, 249
Treatment, of mental illness. See also Medication; Psychiatry; Psychotherapy
adjustment disorders, 86
alcoholism, 134–137
anorexia, 173–174
bipolar disorder, 10–11
body dysmorphic disorder, 110
bulimia, 176
depersonalization disorder, 118
depression, 237, 240
dermatitis, 94
dissociative fugue, 117
dissociative identity disorder, 116
drug abuse, 134–137
generalized anxiety disorder, 109
hypochondriasis, 113
intensive outpatient care, 321
intermittent explosive disorder, 228
loss and, 201
migraines, 93
obesity, 179–181

obsessive-compulsive disorder, 105
panic disorders, 103
partial hospitalization, 321
phobias, 104
posttraumatic stress disorder, 108
psychoses, 15
psychosomatic disorders, 95
psychotic disorders, 272–273
schizophrenia, 261–262, 264–267
sexual disorders, 156–159, 162
social phobia, 104
Tricyclic antidepressants, 246. See also Antidepressants
Trifluoperazine, 261
Trihexyphenidyl, 264
Trilafon, 261
True and False Accusations of Child Abuse (Gardner), 148
Trust-mistrust relationship, and child development, 26–27
Tuberculosis, 247
Tumors, of brain, 277–278, 279, 280–281
Twin studies
of alcoholism, 46
of bipolar disorder, 45
on homosexuality, 161
of panic disorder, 46
of schizophrenia, 44
Tyramine, 247–248

Ulcerative colitis, 90
Ulcers
as psychosomatic illness, 87, 89–90
stress and, 19, 53, 277
Unconscious, theory of, 293–294

Undifferentiated type, of
    schizophrenia, 258
Unemployment. *See also* Work
    adjustment disorders and, 86
    stress and, 63
Urophilia, 152
Urticaria, 93

Vaginismus, 156
Valium, 305
Violence
    influence of media on children
        and adolescents, 48
    intermittent explosive disorder
        and, 229–230
    sadism and history of in family,
        151
Virtues, and Erikson's approach to
    child development, 27
Vitamins, 72
Vivactil, 246
Voyeurism, 152

Weight Watchers groups, 179
Withdrawal, and substance abuse,
    123, 127–128
Women's liberation movement,
    41
Word salad, and schizophrenia,
    255
Work
    loss and issues related to,
        193–194
    mentoring and, 62
    stress and, 3–4, 62–64

Xanax, 103, 305
Xenophobia, 104

Young adult stage, of child
    development, 29–30

Zoloft, 248
Zoophilia, 152–153